As a 59-year-old personal trainer and educational psychologist with a brief background in the military, my life story is one of discipline, resilience, and transformation. I am Sam, and this is my journey.

My Early Years and Military Experience:

 Growing up, I always had a deep-seated drive to excel. I was passionate about sports and outdoor activities, which set the stage for my future. My fascination with discipline and structure led me to enlist in the military at a young age. The military life tested my physical and mental boundaries, teaching me about strength, endurance, and the power of surpassing my limits. It was in the military where I learned the value of teamwork, leadership, and adaptability.

Transitioning to Civilian Life:

After serving with distinction, I transitioned back to civilian life, carrying with me the lessons and values of my military experience. Transitioned into the Offshore diving industry. During periods shore side I discovered my passion for personal training, using my military background to inspire and guide others in their fitness journeys.

 My training approach went beyond physical exercise; I focused on instilling discipline, confidence, and resilience in my clients.

Delving into Educational Psychology:

My curiosity led me to explore the field of educational psychology, enriching my approach to training. This knowledge allowed me to create programs that were mentally engaging and tailored to individual needs, making my training sessions about more than just physical health

My Career as a Personal Trainer:

Now, I use my unique blend of military discipline and psychological insights to help a diverse range of clients. From young athletes to older adults, I guide them in unlocking their potential and transforming their lives.

My Philosophy and Legacy:

At this stage in my life, I firmly believe in the interconnectedness of physical fitness and mental strength. I advocate for a holistic approach to health, emphasizing the importance of self-challenge, goal-setting, and maintaining discipline. My story is not just about physical transformation but about how discipline can shape one's life and destiny. I stand as a testament to what can be achieved through hard work, perseverance, and a profound understanding of the human mind and body.

Table Of Contents

Chapter 1: The Importance of Fitness After 40

The Changing Needs of the Body

As we age, our bodies undergo numerous changes that can impact our overall health and wellness. It is crucial for middle-aged men and women to understand these changes and adapt their fitness and exercise routines accordingly. This subchapter aims to shed light on the changing needs of the body and provide valuable insights for individuals seeking to maintain their physical well-being.

One of the most significant changes that occur with age is a decrease in muscle mass. This can result in a slower metabolism and reduced strength, making it essential to incorporate strength training exercises into your fitness regimen. By engaging in activities such as weightlifting or resistance training, you can help maintain and even increase muscle mass, improving your metabolism and overall physical capability.

Another crucial aspect to consider is flexibility. With age, our joints and muscles tend to become stiffer, which can increase the risk of injuries. Incorporating regular stretching exercises, such as yoga or pilates, can help improve flexibility and enhance mobility. It is important to note that proper form and technique should always be prioritized to prevent strain or injury.

Additionally, the aging process often brings about changes in bone density, making middle-aged individuals more susceptible to osteoporosis and fractures. Weight-bearing exercises, like walking or jogging, can help strengthen bones and reduce the risk of such conditions. It is worth mentioning that consulting with a fitness and exercise wellness coach can provide personalized guidance on the most suitable exercises for your specific needs and goals.

Furthermore, cardiovascular health becomes increasingly important as we age. Regular aerobic exercise, such as swimming or cycling, can help improve heart health, lower blood pressure, and manage weight. Engaging in at least 150 minutes of moderate-intensity aerobic activity every week is recommended to promote overall cardiovascular fitness.

Lastly, it is crucial to address the importance of rest and recovery. As we age, our bodies may require more time to recover from intense physical activity. Adequate rest and sleep are vital for muscle repair and overall well-being. Incorporating relaxation techniques, such as meditation or deep breathing exercises, can also help reduce stress levels and promote overall mental and physical balance.

Understanding and adapting to the changing needs of the body is essential for middle-aged men and women seeking to maintain their fitness and overall well-being. By incorporating strength training, flexibility exercises, weight-bearing activities, aerobic exercise, and sufficient rest, individuals can unleash their full potential, leading a vibrant and healthy life even after 40. Remember, consulting with a fitness and exercise wellness coach can provide valuable guidance and support on your fitness journey.

Common Health Concerns for Middle-Aged Individuals

As we reach our middle-age, our bodies undergo various changes that can impact our overall health and well-being. It is crucial for both men and women in this age group to be aware of the common health concerns they may face and take proactive steps to maintain their fitness and vitality. In this subchapter, we will discuss some of the key health concerns that middle-aged individuals should be mindful of.

1. Cardiovascular Health: Heart disease becomes a prominent concern as we age. Regular exercise, a balanced diet, and stress management techniques can help maintain a healthy heart. It is important to monitor blood pressure and cholesterol levels regularly and consult a healthcare professional for guidance.

2. Musculoskeletal Health: With age, the risk of developing conditions such as osteoporosis and arthritis increases. Engaging in weight-bearing exercises, resistance training, and incorporating calcium-rich foods in the diet can help improve bone density and joint health.

3. Metabolic Health: Middle-aged individuals often experience changes in metabolism, which can lead to weight gain and an increased risk of developing type 2 diabetes. A combination of aerobic exercises, strength training, and a balanced diet can help manage weight and maintain a healthy metabolism.

4. Mental Health: Middle age can bring about various stressors, including career changes, financial responsibilities, and family dynamics. Prioritizing mental well-being is essential. Regular exercise, meditation, and seeking support from loved ones or a mental health professional can help manage stress and promote emotional balance.

5. Hormonal Changes: Both men and women may experience hormonal changes during middle age, including menopause in women and andropause in men. It is important to be aware of the associated symptoms and seek medical advice if necessary.

6. Cancer Prevention: Middle-aged individuals should be diligent about regular screenings for various cancers, such as breast, prostate, and colorectal. Adopting a healthy lifestyle, including a balanced diet rich in fruits and vegetables and avoiding tobacco and excessive alcohol consumption, can significantly reduce the risk of developing cancer.

By understanding and addressing these common health concerns, middle-aged individuals can make informed decisions about their fitness and well-being. Consulting with a fitness and exercise wellness coach can provide additional guidance and support in developing personalized strategies to maintain optimal health in this stage of life. Remember, it is never too late to invest in your health and unleash your potential after 40.

Benefits of Regular Exercise in Midlife

Regular exercise plays a crucial role in maintaining overall health and well-being, particularly in midlife. As we age, our bodies undergo various changes that can impact our physical and mental health. However, incorporating regular exercise into our daily routine can significantly enhance our quality of life and unleash our full potential. In this subchapter, we will explore the numerous benefits that regular exercise offers to middle-aged men and women.

1. Improved physical health: Engaging in regular exercise helps maintain a healthy weight, lowers the risk of chronic diseases such as heart disease, diabetes, and certain types of cancer. It strengthens the cardiovascular system, improves lung function, and enhances bone density, reducing the risk of osteoporosis.

2. Enhanced mental well-being: Exercise has a profound impact on mental health by reducing symptoms of anxiety and depression, boosting mood, and promoting better sleep patterns. Regular physical activity stimulates the production of endorphins, also known as the "feel-good" hormones, increasing overall happiness and reducing stress levels.

3. Increased energy and stamina: Regular exercise improves muscle strength and endurance, leading to increased energy levels and enhanced stamina. Middle-aged individuals who exercise regularly often experience reduced fatigue and are better equipped to handle the demands of daily life.

4. Weight management: As metabolism tends to slow down with age, it becomes increasingly important to maintain a healthy weight. Regular exercise helps burn calories, build lean muscle mass, and increase metabolism, making weight management more attainable.

5. Improved cognitive function: Exercise has been shown to improve cognitive function and memory, reducing the risk of age-related cognitive decline and diseases like dementia. Physical activity stimulates the growth of new brain cells and enhances brain function, promoting mental sharpness and clarity.

6. Social engagement: Engaging in regular exercise provides opportunities for social interaction and connection, which is vital for overall well-being. Joining fitness classes, sports clubs, or exercise groups allows middle-aged individuals to meet new people with similar interests, fostering a sense of community and support.

In conclusion, regular exercise in midlife offers a plethora of benefits, positively impacting both physical and mental health. From improved physical fitness to enhanced mental well-being, the advantages of incorporating exercise into one's routine are undeniable. By prioritizing regular exercise, middle-aged men and women can unleash their full potential, leading healthier, happier, and more fulfilling lives.

In order to achieve optimal physical fitness, it is crucial to have a clear understanding of where you currently stand in terms of your fitness levels. This is where physical fitness assessment tools come into play. These tools are designed to provide valuable insights into your overall fitness and help you set realistic goals for your fitness journey. In this subchapter, we will explore some of the most effective physical fitness assessment tools that can benefit middle-aged men and women looking to improve their fitness levels.

One of the most popular assessment tools is the body composition analysis. This tool helps determine the ratio of fat to lean muscle mass in your body. As we age, the metabolism slows down, and it becomes easier to accumulate excess body fat. By assessing your body composition, you can identify areas that require improvement and tailor your exercise and nutrition plans accordingly.

Another useful assessment tool is the cardiovascular fitness test, which measures your heart's ability to efficiently transport oxygen to your muscles during physical activity. As middle-aged individuals, maintaining good cardiovascular health is essential for overall well-being. By assessing your cardiovascular fitness, you can identify any potential areas of concern and work towards improving your heart health.

Flexibility is another important aspect of physical fitness, especially as we age. Therefore, incorporating a flexibility assessment tool is crucial. This tool measures your range of motion and identifies any areas of stiffness or tightness in your joints and muscles. By working on improving your flexibility, you can reduce the risk of injuries and enhance your overall performance during exercise.

Finally, it is crucial to assess your muscular strength and endurance. Strength training becomes even more important as we age, as it helps maintain muscle mass and bone density. By utilizing a strength and endurance assessment tool, you can determine your current strength levels and create a targeted strength training program to gradually improve your muscular fitness.

By utilizing these physical fitness assessment tools, middle-aged men and women can gain valuable insights into their current fitness levels and set realistic goals for their fitness journey. It is important to consult with a fitness and exercise wellness coach who can guide you through the assessment process and help you interpret the results. Remember, everyone's fitness journey is unique, and a personalized approach is key to unleashing your potential after 40.

Understanding Your Body Composition

In order to achieve optimal fitness and overall wellness, it is crucial to understand your body composition. Middle-aged men and women often face unique challenges when it comes to maintaining a healthy lifestyle, as age-related changes can impact body composition and overall health. By understanding the key components of body composition, you can develop effective strategies to unleash your potential and achieve your fitness goals.

Body composition refers to the proportion of different components that make up your body, including fat, muscle, bone, and water. Traditionally, weight alone has been used as a measure of health and fitness, but this fails to consider the distribution of weight and the ratio of fat to muscle. For middle-aged individuals, this is particularly important, as the body tends to undergo changes that affect body composition. These changes include a decrease in muscle mass and an increase in body fat, both of which can have negative implications for overall health.

By understanding your body composition, you can gain insights into how to improve your fitness and well-being. For instance, if you discover that you have a high percentage of body fat, it may be an indication that you need to focus on losing fat and increasing muscle mass. On the other hand, if you have a low percentage of body fat but limited muscle mass, you may need to prioritize strength training exercises to build lean muscle.

Measuring body composition can be done through various methods, such as skinfold calipers, bioelectrical impedance, or dual-energy X-ray absorptiometry (DEXA) scans. These methods provide valuable information about your body fat percentage, muscle mass, and overall health. Consulting with a fitness and exercise wellness coach can help you understand and interpret these measurements, providing you with personalized recommendations to improve your body composition.

Incorporating a balanced exercise routine and a healthy diet are essential for optimizing body composition. Strength training exercises can help increase muscle mass, boost metabolism, and decrease body fat. Cardiovascular activities are also important for improving heart health and promoting fat loss. Additionally, consuming a nutrient-rich diet that includes lean proteins, whole grains, fruits, and vegetables can support muscle growth and help maintain a healthy weight.

In conclusion, understanding your body composition is crucial for middle-aged men and women looking to improve their fitness and overall wellness. By assessing your body fat percentage, muscle mass, and overall health, you can develop a personalized plan to optimize your body composition. Through a combination of strength training, cardiovascular exercises, and a healthy diet, you can unleash your potential and achieve the fitness goals you desire. Consulting with a fitness and exercise wellness coach can provide you with the guidance and support needed to navigate the journey towards improved body composition and a healthier lifestyle.

Evaluating Cardiovascular Endurance

In the pursuit of a healthy and active lifestyle, cardiovascular endurance plays a crucial role. It refers to the ability of the heart, lungs, and blood vessels to supply oxygen and nutrients to the working muscles efficiently. As we age, our cardiovascular system naturally undergoes changes, making it essential for middle-aged men and women to evaluate their cardiovascular endurance regularly. By doing so, they can gauge their fitness levels, set realistic goals, and make necessary adjustments to their exercise routines.

There are several effective methods to evaluate cardiovascular endurance. One common approach is the use of a submaximal exercise test, such as the 1.5-mile walk or the 12-minute run. These tests measure the time it takes to complete a specific distance or the distance covered within a set time frame. By analyzing the results, fitness and exercise wellness coaches can assess an individual's cardiovascular fitness level and determine if any improvements are needed.

Additionally, heart rate monitoring is a valuable tool in evaluating cardiovascular endurance. During exercise, the heart rate increases to meet the body's oxygen demands. By monitoring heart rate before, during, and after physical activity, individuals can gain insight into their cardiovascular fitness. Fitness trackers and smartwatches equipped with heart rate monitors are widely available and provide real-time feedback, making it easier for middle-aged men and women to assess their cardiovascular endurance during workouts.

Another useful method is the talk test, which requires no equipment. It involves assessing an individual's ability to carry on a conversation while exercising. If one can comfortably speak in full sentences during moderate-intensity activities, it indicates good cardiovascular endurance. However, if breathlessness hinders speech or results in short, choppy sentences, it may suggest a need to improve cardiovascular fitness.

Furthermore, the 6-Minute Walk Test is a simple yet effective way to evaluate cardiovascular endurance. It measures the distance covered by individuals within six minutes of walking at their own pace. This test provides valuable information about aerobic capacity and can be easily conducted in a variety of settings.

Regularly evaluating cardiovascular endurance allows middle-aged men and women to track their progress and make informed decisions about their fitness journey. By consulting with a fitness and exercise wellness coach, individuals can receive guidance on appropriate exercises, training intensity, and potential adjustments to improve cardiovascular endurance. Remember, the key to unleashing your potential after 40 lies in understanding and optimizing your cardiovascular health.

Assessing Muscular Strength and Flexibility

As we age, it becomes even more crucial to prioritize our overall health and well-being. Regular exercise not only helps us maintain a healthy weight, but it also plays a vital role in preserving muscular strength and flexibility. In this subchapter, we will explore the importance of assessing your muscular strength and flexibility, and how these assessments can guide your fitness journey towards unleashing your potential after 40.

Muscular strength is the ability of your muscles to exert force against resistance. It is an essential component of overall fitness, enabling you to perform daily activities with ease and reducing the risk of injuries. Assessing your muscular strength can help you determine your current fitness level and set realistic goals for improvement. This can be done through various tests, such as the one-repetition maximum (1RM) test or the handgrip strength test. These assessments provide valuable information about your muscle strength and help you track your progress over time.

Flexibility, on the other hand, refers to the range of motion in your joints and muscles. Maintaining good flexibility is crucial for performing everyday tasks, preventing muscle imbalances, and reducing the risk of injuries. Assessing your flexibility can be done through simple tests like the sit-and-reach test or shoulder flexibility test. By understanding your current level of flexibility, you can tailor your exercise routine to focus on stretching and mobility exercises that target specific areas of improvement.

For middle-aged men and women, it is essential to work with a fitness and exercise wellness coach who can guide you through the assessment process. These professionals have the knowledge and expertise to conduct accurate assessments and design personalized workout programs based on your specific needs and goals. They can help you identify any muscular imbalances or limitations that may hinder your progress and provide appropriate exercises and modifications to address them.

Regular assessments of muscular strength and flexibility are key to monitoring your progress and adjusting your fitness routine accordingly. As we age, our bodies change, and it is important to adapt our exercise program to accommodate those changes. By regularly assessing your muscular strength and flexibility, you can ensure that you are maximizing your potential and maintaining optimal health and wellness.

In conclusion, assessing muscular strength and flexibility is crucial for middle-aged men and women seeking to improve their fitness and unleash their potential after 40. These assessments provide valuable insights into your current fitness level, help set realistic goals, and enable you to track your progress. Working with a fitness and exercise wellness coach ensures that you receive personalized guidance and support throughout your fitness journey. By prioritizing regular assessments, you can optimize your workouts, address any limitations, and lead a healthier, more active lifestyle.

Chapter 3: Designing an Effective Exercise Program

Setting Realistic Goals

In the journey towards leading a healthier and more fulfilling life, setting realistic goals is a crucial step for middle-aged men and women. As a fitness and exercise wellness coach, it is essential to guide individuals in understanding the importance of setting achievable targets to avoid disappointment and maintain motivation.

The first aspect to consider when setting goals is to ensure they are realistic and attainable. Middle-aged individuals often have various responsibilities and commitments, such as family, career, and personal life, which can make it challenging to dedicate extensive time to fitness. Therefore, it is vital to set goals that are manageable within their current lifestyle. Encourage them to start small, gradually increasing the intensity and duration of their workouts as they progress. This will prevent burnout and decrease the chances of injury or frustration.

Another crucial element is to promote a holistic approach to goal setting. While physical fitness is undoubtedly important, it is equally essential to consider other aspects of wellness, such as mental and emotional health. Encourage individuals to set goals that encompass all these dimensions, such as incorporating stress management techniques, improving sleep quality, or practicing mindfulness. This comprehensive approach not only ensures overall well-being but also increases the chances of sustained success in achieving their goals.

Furthermore, it is essential to emphasize the significance of tracking progress. Encourage middle-aged men and women to keep a record of their workouts, dietary choices, and any other relevant information. This tracking system will help them identify patterns, make necessary adjustments, and stay motivated by witnessing their progress over time. Remind them that progress is not always linear, and setbacks are a natural part of the journey. It is crucial to view setbacks as learning opportunities and not as reasons to give up.

Lastly, as a fitness and exercise wellness coach, it is essential to instill a sense of self-compassion and flexibility in goal setting. Middle-aged individuals may face unique challenges, such as physical limitations or health concerns. Encourage them to adapt their goals accordingly and always prioritize their well-being above all else. Remind them that the ultimate goal is to lead a healthier and happier life, and it is not a race against time or an opportunity to compare oneself to others.

In conclusion, setting realistic goals is a fundamental step for middle-aged individuals in their pursuit of a healthier lifestyle. As a fitness and exercise wellness coach, guide them in understanding the importance of attainable goals, a holistic approach, tracking progress, and self-compassion. By adopting these principles, middle-aged men and women can unleash their potential and achieve long-term success in their fitness journey.

Choosing the Right Types of Exercise

When it comes to maintaining fitness and wellness after 40, choosing the right types of exercise becomes increasingly important. As middle-aged men and women, our bodies undergo various changes, and it is crucial to adapt our exercise routines accordingly. In this subchapter, we will explore the key factors to consider when selecting exercises that best suit your needs and goals.

One vital aspect to keep in mind is the importance of cardiovascular exercise. Engaging in activities that elevate your heart rate not only improves cardiovascular health but also aids in weight management and reduces the risk of chronic diseases such as heart disease and diabetes. Options such as brisk walking, swimming, cycling, or dancing are excellent choices for middle-aged individuals who want to improve their cardiovascular fitness without putting excessive strain on their joints.

Strength training exercises are equally crucial for maintaining muscle mass and bone density as we age. Incorporating resistance training into your routine helps to increase muscle strength and improve overall body composition. Exercises utilizing free weights, resistance bands, or machines can be tailored to your fitness level and personal goals. Additionally, strength training has been shown to enhance metabolism, making it an effective tool for weight management.

Flexibility exercises should not be overlooked, as they play a vital role in maintaining joint health and preventing injuries. As we age, our muscles and tendons become less pliable, increasing the risk of strains and sprains. Yoga, Pilates, and stretching exercises are excellent choices for middle-aged individuals, as they improve flexibility, balance, and posture.

Lastly, it is essential to consider your personal preferences and lifestyle when choosing the right types of exercise. Engaging in activities that you genuinely enjoy will increase the likelihood of adherence and long-term success. Whether it's joining a local sports team, taking up a dance class, or hiking in nature, finding activities that bring you joy will make your fitness journey more enjoyable and sustainable.

As a fitness and exercise wellness coach, I encourage all middle-aged men and women to prioritize their health and well-being by selecting the right types of exercise. A well-rounded routine incorporating cardiovascular, strength training, and flexibility exercises will help you maximize your potential and unlock a healthier, more fulfilling life after 40. Remember, it's never too late to invest in yourself and unleash your true potential.

Creating a Balanced Workout Routine

In order to achieve optimal health and fitness goals, it is essential to establish a well-rounded and balanced workout routine. This subchapter will guide middle-aged men and women towards creating a personalized exercise plan that caters to their specific needs and goals. As a fitness and exercise wellness coach, it is crucial to understand the importance of balance in a workout routine, considering the unique challenges that individuals in this age group may face.

Firstly, it is essential to incorporate a combination of cardiovascular exercises, strength training, and flexibility exercises into the workout routine. Cardiovascular exercises such as brisk walking, jogging, swimming, or cycling help to improve heart health, boost metabolism, and burn calories. Strength training exercises, on the other hand, are crucial for building lean muscle mass, increasing bone density, and enhancing overall strength. This can be achieved through resistance training, weightlifting, or even bodyweight exercises. Flexibility exercises such as yoga or stretching routines aid in improving joint mobility, preventing injuries, and enhancing overall flexibility.

When creating a balanced workout routine, it is important to take into consideration individual goals and limitations. For example, if weight loss is a primary goal, focusing on a combination of cardiovascular exercises and strength training will be beneficial. On the other hand, if building strength and improving flexibility are the main objectives, incorporating more strength training and flexibility exercises into the routine is recommended.

Additionally, it is crucial to vary the intensity and duration of workouts to prevent boredom and ensure continual progress. Incorporating high-intensity interval training (HIIT) or circuit training can significantly boost cardiovascular fitness while saving time. On the other hand, low-intensity workouts, such as gentle yoga or walking, can provide active recovery periods and aid in relaxation.

Lastly, it is important to allow for adequate rest and recovery between workouts. This can be achieved by scheduling rest days or incorporating active recovery days, such as light stretching or yoga sessions. Rest and recovery are crucial for preventing overtraining, reducing the risk of injuries, and allowing the body to adapt and grow stronger.

In conclusion, creating a balanced workout routine is essential for middle-aged men and women to achieve optimal health and fitness. As a fitness and exercise wellness coach, it is important to assist individuals in developing a personalized plan that combines cardiovascular exercises, strength training, and flexibility exercises. By considering individual goals and limitations, varying the intensity and duration of workouts, and allowing for proper rest and recovery, individuals can unleash their potential and enjoy a healthy and active lifestyle.

Incorporating Cardiovascular Training

Cardiovascular training, often referred to as cardio, is a fundamental component of any fitness regimen. It is especially crucial for middle-aged men and women who are looking to maintain or improve their overall health and well-being. In this subchapter, we will explore the importance of cardiovascular training and provide practical tips on how to incorporate it into your exercise routine.

First and foremost, cardiovascular training is essential for maintaining a healthy heart and circulatory system. As we age, our cardiovascular system becomes less efficient, making us more susceptible to heart disease and other related conditions. Regular cardio exercises, such as running, cycling, swimming, or brisk walking, can help strengthen the heart muscle, lower blood pressure, and improve blood circulation, reducing the risk of developing cardiovascular diseases.

Moreover, cardio workouts aid in weight management and can assist middle-aged individuals in maintaining a healthy body weight. As our metabolism slows down with age, it becomes easier to gain weight and harder to shed those extra pounds. Engaging in cardiovascular exercises allows you to burn calories, improve metabolism, and maintain a healthy body composition.

When incorporating cardiovascular training into your exercise routine, it is essential to start gradually and progress at your own pace. If you have not been physically active for a while or have any underlying medical conditions, it is recommended to consult with a fitness and exercise wellness coach before embarking on a new cardio regimen.

To make cardiovascular training more enjoyable and sustainable, try incorporating a variety of exercises into your routine. Mixing different activities, such as jogging, cycling, and swimming, not only keeps your workouts interesting but also engages different muscle groups and prevents overuse injuries.

Additionally, consider integrating high-intensity interval training (HIIT) into your cardiovascular workouts. HIIT involves alternating short bursts of intense activity with periods of rest or light activity. This type of training has been shown to be highly effective in improving cardiovascular fitness, burning calories, and boosting metabolism.

Lastly, do not forget to listen to your body and take rest days when needed. Overtraining can lead to injuries and burnout, so it is crucial to find a balance between challenging yourself and allowing your body to recover.

Incorporating cardiovascular training into your fitness routine is a fantastic way to improve your overall health and unleash your potential after 40. By engaging in regular cardio exercises, you can strengthen your heart, manage your weight, and enhance your well-being. Remember to start slowly, mix up your workouts, and listen to your body. With dedication and consistency, you will reap the countless benefits of cardiovascular training for years to come.

Focusing on Strength and Resistance Training

As we age, it becomes increasingly important to prioritize our fitness and overall well-being. Strength and resistance training are two key components that can significantly improve our physical health, mental well-being, and overall quality of life. In this subchapter, we will delve into the benefits and strategies of incorporating strength and resistance training into your fitness routine.

For middle-aged men and women, strength and resistance training offer a multitude of advantages. Not only does it help increase muscle mass and bone density, but it also boosts metabolism, enhances joint stability, and improves overall body composition. Engaging in regular strength training exercises can also reduce the risk of developing chronic conditions such as osteoporosis, heart disease, and diabetes.

To maximize the benefits of strength and resistance training, it is essential to work with a fitness and exercise wellness coach who can tailor a program to your individual needs and goals. These professionals possess the expertise to develop a plan that suits your fitness level, takes into account any existing health conditions, and ensures proper form and technique to prevent injuries.

When it comes to strength training, a combination of resistance exercises using free weights, machines, or bodyweight can be highly effective. By gradually increasing the intensity and resistance over time, you can continually challenge your muscles and promote growth. Examples of strength training exercises include squats, deadlifts, bench presses, and push-ups.

Resistance training, on the other hand, focuses on using various resistance tools such as resistance bands or cables to build strength. This type of training targets specific muscle groups and can be particularly beneficial for improving muscular endurance and flexibility. Incorporating exercises like bicep curls, tricep extensions, and lateral raises into your routine can help you achieve a well-rounded workout.

Remember, consistency is key when it comes to strength and resistance training. Aim for at least two to three sessions per week, allowing your body time to recover between workouts. It is also crucial to listen to your body and adjust the intensity and duration of your exercises as necessary.

In conclusion, middle-aged men and women can greatly benefit from incorporating strength and resistance training into their fitness journey. By working with a fitness and exercise wellness coach, you can develop a customized program that addresses your unique needs and goals. Remember to start slowly, progress gradually, and stay committed to reaping the countless rewards that come with increasing your strength and overall fitness.

Enhancing Flexibility and Mobility

As we age, maintaining flexibility and mobility becomes increasingly important for our overall health and wellbeing. In this subchapter, we will explore various strategies and exercises to help you enhance your flexibility and mobility, allowing you to lead a more active and fulfilling life.

Flexibility is the ability of our muscles and joints to move through their full range of motion. It is crucial for performing daily activities, such as bending, reaching, and even tying our shoelaces. By incorporating regular flexibility exercises into your fitness routine, you can improve your posture, reduce the risk of injury, and enhance your athletic performance.

One effective way to enhance flexibility is through stretching exercises. Dynamic stretching, which involves moving parts of your body through a full range of motion, is ideal for warming up before exercise. It helps increase blood flow to the muscles, preparing them for the physical exertion to come. Static stretching, on the other hand, involves holding a stretch for a certain period, and it is best done after physical activity to help relax and lengthen the muscles.

In addition to stretching, mobility exercises play a vital role in maintaining healthy joints and muscles. These exercises focus on improving the range of motion in specific joints, such as the hips, shoulders, and spine. By incorporating mobility exercises into your fitness routine, you can alleviate joint stiffness, enhance balance, and even reduce the risk of falls.

Some effective mobility exercises include shoulder rotations, hip circles, and spinal twists. These exercises can be done with or without equipment, making them accessible and convenient for everyone. Remember to start slowly and gradually increase the intensity and duration of your exercises to avoid strain or injury.

As a fitness and exercise wellness coach, it is important to emphasize the importance of consistency and patience when working towards enhancing flexibility and mobility. Results may not be immediate, but with regular practice, you will start to notice improvements in your range of motion and overall physical functioning.

In conclusion, enhancing flexibility and mobility is essential for middle-aged men and women who want to maintain an active and fulfilling lifestyle. By incorporating stretching and mobility exercises into your fitness routine, you can improve your posture, reduce the risk of injury, and enhance your overall quality of life. Remember, it's never too late to start prioritizing your flexibility and mobility – your body will thank you for it!

Chapter 4: Nutrition and Diet for Optimal Fitness

Understanding the Role of Nutrition in Fitness

Proper nutrition is an essential component of any fitness journey, especially for middle-aged men and women who are looking to unleash their potential after 40. In this subchapter, we will delve into the significance of nutrition in achieving optimal fitness and provide valuable insights for fitness and exercise wellness coaches working with this specific audience.

As we age, our bodies undergo various changes, including a decrease in muscle mass, slower metabolism, and hormonal fluctuations. These factors make it even more crucial to pay attention to our nutritional intake to support our fitness goals and overall well-being.

First and foremost, it is important to emphasize the importance of a balanced diet. Middle-aged individuals should focus on consuming a variety of nutrient-dense foods that provide the necessary vitamins, minerals, and macronutrients. This includes incorporating lean proteins, whole grains, fruits, vegetables, and healthy fats into their meals. A balanced diet not only fuels the body but also aids in muscle recovery and growth.

Furthermore, middle-aged men and women should be mindful of their caloric intake. As metabolism tends to slow down with age, it is essential to adjust calorie consumption accordingly to maintain a healthy weight. This can be achieved by understanding individual energy needs and finding the right balance between calories consumed and calories burned through physical activity.

In addition to a balanced diet, hydration plays a crucial role in fitness and overall health. Middle-aged individuals should prioritize drinking an adequate amount of water throughout the day, as dehydration can lead to decreased performance, muscle cramps, and fatigue.

Lastly, it is essential to address the importance of personalized nutrition plans. Fitness and exercise wellness coaches working with middle-aged individuals should take into account their specific goals, health conditions, and dietary preferences when designing nutrition plans. By tailoring these plans to individual needs, coaches can help their clients achieve maximum results and maintain long-term success.

In conclusion, nutrition is an integral part of any fitness journey, particularly for middle-aged men and women. By understanding the role of nutrition, individuals can unlock their full potential after 40. Fitness and exercise wellness coaches play a vital role in guiding and supporting this demographic, providing them with the knowledge and tools to make informed dietary choices and optimize their overall fitness levels.

Balancing Macronutrients for Energy

In the quest for optimal health and fitness, one aspect that often gets overlooked is the importance of balancing macronutrients for energy. As we age, our bodies undergo various changes that can impact our energy levels and overall well-being. Middle-aged men and women, who are seeking to unleash their potential after 40, can greatly benefit from understanding and implementing a macronutrient-balanced diet.

Macronutrients, which include carbohydrates, proteins, and fats, are the primary sources of energy for our bodies. Each of these macronutrients plays a crucial role in maintaining our physical and mental health. However, the key lies in finding the right balance that suits our individual needs and goals.

Carbohydrates are the body's preferred source of energy. They provide us with the fuel needed to perform daily activities and exercise. Whole grains, fruits, and vegetables are excellent sources of complex carbohydrates that provide sustained energy and essential nutrients. Middle-aged individuals should focus on incorporating these into their diet while monitoring their portion sizes to avoid excessive carbohydrate consumption.

Proteins are the building blocks of our bodies. They aid in muscle repair and growth, support immune function, and contribute to overall well-being. Lean meats, fish, eggs, legumes, and dairy products are excellent sources of protein. Middle-aged men and women should aim to include a variety of protein sources in their meals to ensure they meet their daily requirements.

Fats, often misunderstood, are crucial for our body's proper functioning. Healthy fats, such as those found in avocados, nuts, seeds, and olive oil, provide a steady source of energy and support brain health. Middle-aged individuals should opt for unsaturated fats over saturated and trans fats, which can have negative effects on heart health.

Achieving a macronutrient balance is not about strict diets or deprivation but rather about making informed choices. Consulting a fitness and exercise wellness coach can provide valuable guidance in creating a personalized nutrition plan. They can help middle-aged individuals understand their specific needs, set realistic goals, and make sustainable changes to their eating habits.

In conclusion, balancing macronutrients for energy is a crucial aspect of unleashing one's potential after 40. Middle-aged men and women should prioritize a diet that includes a balance of carbohydrates, proteins, and healthy fats. By doing so, they can optimize their energy levels, improve their overall well-being, and make significant strides towards their fitness and health goals.

Incorporating Micronutrients for Overall Health

As we age, our bodies undergo various changes that can impact our overall health and well-being. One crucial aspect of maintaining optimal health is ensuring that we receive adequate amounts of essential micronutrients. Micronutrients are vitamins and minerals that our bodies require in small quantities but play a significant role in supporting our overall health and longevity.

Middle-aged men and women often face unique challenges when it comes to maintaining their fitness and overall health. Hormonal changes, decreased metabolic rate, and increased risk of chronic diseases can all take a toll on their well-being. However, by incorporating micronutrients into their diet, they can counteract these effects and unleash their full potential.

Vitamins and minerals are essential for a wide range of bodily functions. They support the immune system, promote healthy cell growth and repair, and help maintain optimal energy levels. Including a variety of fruits, vegetables, whole grains, and lean proteins in your diet can provide you with the necessary micronutrients to support these functions.

Certain micronutrients are particularly important for middle-aged individuals. Calcium and vitamin D, for example, are crucial for maintaining bone health and reducing the risk of osteoporosis. As our bodies age, our bones become more brittle and susceptible to fractures. By ensuring an adequate intake of calcium-rich foods such as dairy products, leafy greens, and fortified cereals, and getting enough sun exposure for vitamin D synthesis, middle-aged men and women can protect their bone health and overall well-being.

Another essential micronutrient for middle-aged individuals is vitamin B12. This vitamin is necessary for the production of red blood cells and the proper functioning of the nervous system. As we age, our bodies become less efficient at absorbing B12 from food sources. Therefore, it is crucial to incorporate B12-rich foods such as meat, fish, eggs, and dairy products into your diet. If necessary, supplements can also be considered, under the guidance of a healthcare professional.

Incorporating micronutrients into your diet can have a profound impact on your overall health and well-being. By focusing on a balanced diet that includes a variety of nutrient-dense foods, you can ensure that your body receives the essential vitamins and minerals it needs to function optimally. Consult with a fitness and exercise wellness coach to develop a personalized nutrition plan that meets your specific needs. Remember, it's never too late to start prioritizing your health and unleashing your potential after 40.

Hydration and Its Impact on Performance

Staying properly hydrated is crucial for individuals of all ages, but as we age, the importance of hydration becomes even more significant. In this subchapter, we will explore the vital role that hydration plays in enhancing performance and overall wellness for middle-aged men and women. As fitness and exercise wellness coaches, it is essential for us to understand the direct impact of hydration on our clients' progress and success.

Hydration is not just about drinking water; it encompasses the balance between fluid intake and loss. As we age, our bodies become less efficient at regulating water balance, making it more challenging to stay adequately hydrated. This can result in decreased performance, reduced endurance, and increased risk of injuries during exercise.

When it comes to physical performance, hydration has a direct impact on energy levels, muscle function, and cognitive abilities. Dehydration can lead to fatigue, muscle cramps, dizziness, and decreased concentration, all of which can hinder our ability to perform at our best. Middle-aged individuals, who may already face age-related declines in physical fitness, need to be especially conscious of their hydration status to optimize their performance.

Moreover, hydration plays a significant role in maintaining joint health and preventing injuries. Proper hydration helps lubricate the joints, allowing for smooth movement and reducing the risk of joint-related issues such as arthritis. By ensuring adequate hydration, middle-aged men and women can protect their joints and sustain their exercise routines without debilitating pain or discomfort.

In addition to physical performance, hydration also impacts our overall wellness and vitality. Proper hydration supports healthy digestion, aids in nutrient absorption, and helps regulate body temperature. It also promotes healthy skin, reduces the risk of urinary tract infections, and supports kidney function. By prioritizing hydration, middle-aged individuals can improve their overall health and well-being, allowing them to lead active and fulfilling lives.

As fitness and exercise wellness coaches, it is our responsibility to educate our clients about the significance of hydration and guide them in adopting healthy hydration habits. We should emphasize the importance of drinking water throughout the day, particularly before, during, and after exercise. Encouraging the consumption of fruits and vegetables with high water content can also contribute to meeting hydration needs. By understanding and addressing the impact of hydration on performance, we can help middle-aged men and women unleash their full potential and achieve their fitness goals.

As we age, our bodies undergo various changes, and it becomes increasingly important to prioritize our health and well-being. One crucial aspect of maintaining a healthy lifestyle is adopting proper eating habits. In this subchapter, we will explore some effective strategies for healthy eating after the age of 40, specifically tailored to the needs of middle-aged men and women.

1. Prioritize Nutrient-Dense Foods: As we age, our bodies require more nutrients to function optimally. Focus on incorporating nutrient-dense foods into your diet, such as fruits, vegetables, lean proteins, whole grains, and healthy fats. These foods provide essential vitamins, minerals, and antioxidants that promote overall health and longevity.

2. Mindful Eating: Practice mindful eating by slowing down and savoring each bite. Pay attention to your body's hunger and fullness cues, and avoid mindless snacking. This approach can help prevent overeating and promote better digestion.

3. Hydration is Key: Adequate hydration is crucial for maintaining optimal health. As you age, your body's thirst mechanism may become less efficient, so make a conscious effort to drink enough water throughout the day. Aim for at least eight glasses of water daily and limit sugary drinks.

4. Portion Control: Middle age often brings changes in metabolism, making weight management more challenging. Be mindful of portion sizes to avoid consuming excess calories. Use smaller plates and bowls to help control portion sizes, and listen to your body's signals of fullness.

5. Meal Planning and Preparation: Plan your meals in advance to ensure a balanced diet. This practice helps you make healthier choices and prevents impulsive decisions. Dedicate time each week for meal preparation, batch cooking, and storing meals in portioned containers for convenience.

6. Reduce Sodium and Sugar Intake: Excessive sodium and sugar consumption can lead to various health issues, including high blood pressure and diabetes. Read food labels carefully and opt for low-sodium and low-sugar alternatives. Flavor your meals with herbs and spices instead of salt, and satisfy your sweet tooth with natural sugars from fruits.

7. Seek Professional Guidance: Consulting with a fitness and exercise wellness coach can provide valuable insight and personalized guidance for your specific needs. They can help create a customized meal plan, address any nutritional deficiencies, and support you in achieving your health goals.

Remember, healthy eating is a lifelong commitment, and it's never too late to start making positive changes. By implementing these strategies into your daily routine, you can unlock your true potential and enjoy a vibrant and fulfilling life after 40.

Addressing Common Dietary Challenges

As we age, our dietary needs and challenges undergo significant changes. Middle-aged men and women often find themselves struggling with weight management, energy levels, and maintaining overall health. However, with the right knowledge and approach, these challenges can be effectively addressed, allowing you to enjoy a healthy and fulfilling life.

1. Weight Management:

One of the most common dietary challenges faced by middle-aged individuals is weight gain. Hormonal changes, a slower metabolism, and a sedentary lifestyle can all contribute to this. To combat weight gain, it's important to focus on portion control, choose nutrient-dense foods, and avoid processed and sugary foods. Incorporating regular exercise, such as strength training and cardiovascular activities, can also aid in weight management.

2. Energy Levels:

Many middle-aged individuals struggle with low energy levels throughout the day. To address this challenge, it is crucial to make mindful dietary choices. Opt for a balanced diet of whole grains, lean proteins, fruits, and vegetables. Additionally, staying hydrated and avoiding excessive caffeine consumption can help maintain optimal energy levels. Regular exercise and adequate sleep are also vital in boosting energy levels.

3. Maintaining Overall Health:

As we age, our bodies become more susceptible to chronic diseases such as heart disease, diabetes, and osteoporosis. A healthy diet plays a key role in preventing these conditions and maintaining overall health. Include foods rich in vitamins, minerals, and antioxidants, such as leafy greens, colorful fruits, fatty fish, and nuts. Additionally, reducing sodium and saturated fat intake while increasing fiber consumption can significantly improve your health.

4. Healthy Aging:

Middle-aged individuals often face concerns related to aging gracefully and maintaining a youthful appearance. While diet alone cannot reverse the aging process, it can support healthy aging. Include foods high in antioxidants, such as berries and dark chocolate, to combat free radicals and promote skin health. Healthy fats found in avocados, olive oil, and nuts can also contribute to a youthful appearance by nourishing the skin from within.

Remember that addressing common dietary challenges is not about extreme diets or quick fixes. It's about making sustainable lifestyle changes that can be maintained in the long run. Consult with a fitness and exercise wellness coach who can guide you in creating a personalized nutrition plan and offer support throughout your fitness journey. With dedication and proper guidance, you can overcome these challenges, unleash your potential, and embrace a healthier and more fulfilling life after 40.

Chapter 5: Overcoming Obstacles and Staying Motivated

Dealing with Time Constraints and Busy Schedules

In today's fast-paced world, it can be challenging to find time for ourselves, especially when it comes to fitness and exercise. Middle-aged men and women often find themselves overwhelmed by work responsibilities, family obligations, and other commitments, leaving little room for prioritizing their own well-being. However, it is crucial to understand that taking care of our physical and mental health should never be compromised, no matter how busy our schedules may be.

To overcome time constraints and make fitness a priority, it is essential to adopt a strategic approach. As a fitness and exercise wellness coach, I have witnessed countless success stories from men and women who have managed to find the time and achieve their health goals. Here are some practical tips to help you unleash your potential after 40:

1. Prioritize and schedule: Take a close look at your daily routine and identify areas where you can make time for exercise. Block out specific time slots on your calendar dedicated solely to your fitness activities. Treat these appointments as non-negotiable, just like any other important commitment.

2. Time-efficient workouts: When time is limited, focus on high-intensity workouts that deliver maximum results in a shorter period. Interval training, circuit training, or even a quick 20-minute HIIT session can be highly effective in boosting your fitness levels.

3. Incorporate physical activity into your daily routine: Look for opportunities to be active throughout the day. Take the stairs instead of the elevator, walk or bike to work if feasible, or squeeze in short bursts of exercise during breaks.

4. Utilize available resources: If finding time to hit the gym is a challenge, explore options like home workouts, online fitness programs, or fitness apps that offer guided exercises and meal plans. These resources can provide flexibility and convenience, allowing you to exercise whenever and wherever suits your schedule.

5. Make it a family affair: Engage your loved ones in your fitness journey. Plan activities that involve the entire family, such as hiking, biking, or playing sports together. This not only allows you to spend quality time with your family but also encourages everyone to prioritize their well-being.

Remember that consistency is key when it comes to fitness. Even small, regular efforts can yield significant results over time. By effectively managing your time constraints and busy schedules, you can unleash your potential after 40 and experience a healthier, more fulfilling life. Prioritize your own well-being, and watch as it positively impacts every other aspect of your life.

Managing Stress and Balancing Priorities

In today's fast-paced world, managing stress and balancing priorities has become increasingly important, especially for middle-aged men and women. As we age, the responsibilities and demands of life tend to multiply, making it crucial to find effective strategies to maintain our physical and mental well-being. This subchapter aims to provide valuable insights and practical tips to help individuals navigate the challenges of stress management and prioritize their health and fitness goals.

1. Recognizing the Signs of Stress: It is essential to identify the signs of stress early on to prevent its negative impact on our health. This section will discuss common symptoms such as irritability, fatigue, and sleep disturbances. By understanding these warning signs, individuals can take proactive measures to alleviate stress before it overwhelms them.

2. Finding Balance: Balancing priorities is key to maintaining a healthy lifestyle. This section will explore strategies for managing work, family, and personal commitments effectively. It will emphasize the importance of setting boundaries, learning to say no, and delegating tasks to reduce overwhelm and create more time for self-care.

3. Stress-Reducing Techniques: This part of the subchapter will delve into various stress-relieving techniques that can be easily incorporated into daily routines. It will explore practices such as mindfulness meditation, deep breathing exercises, and engaging in hobbies or activities that bring joy and relaxation. These techniques can help middle-aged men and women find solace amidst the chaos of everyday life.

4. Prioritizing Exercise and Fitness: Regular physical activity plays a vital role in managing stress and promoting overall well-being. This section will highlight the significance of exercise for middle-aged individuals and provide practical tips for incorporating fitness into their busy schedules. It will explore different types of exercise, such as strength training, cardiovascular workouts, and flexibility exercises, tailored to their specific needs and abilities.

5. Seeking Professional Guidance: Lastly, this subchapter will emphasize the importance of seeking the expertise of a fitness and exercise wellness coach. These professionals can provide personalized guidance, support, and accountability to help middle-aged men and women overcome obstacles, set realistic goals, and achieve optimal health and fitness.

In conclusion, managing stress and balancing priorities is crucial for middle-aged men and women to live fulfilling and healthy lives. By recognizing stress, finding balance, adopting stress-reducing techniques, prioritizing exercise, and seeking professional guidance, individuals can unleash their potential and unlock their best selves after 40.

Overcoming Age-Related Challenges

As we age, we often find ourselves facing new and unique challenges when it comes to maintaining our health and fitness. However, it is important to remember that age should not be a barrier to achieving our potential and living a fulfilling and active life. In this subchapter, we will explore some of the common age-related challenges that middle-aged men and women may encounter, and discuss strategies for overcoming them.

One of the most common challenges that people face as they get older is a decline in muscle mass and strength. This can make it more difficult to perform everyday tasks and activities, and may lead to an increased risk of injury. However, by incorporating regular strength training exercises into your fitness routine, you can help to maintain and even increase your muscle mass and strength. Working with a fitness and exercise wellness coach can provide you with the guidance and support needed to create a personalized strength training program that suits your individual needs.

Another challenge that many middle-aged individuals face is a decrease in flexibility and mobility. This can make it harder to perform certain exercises and activities, and may increase the risk of developing joint pain or injuries. To overcome this challenge, it is important to prioritize flexibility training in your fitness routine. Incorporating activities such as yoga or Pilates can help to improve your flexibility and range of motion, making it easier to move and perform everyday tasks.

As we age, our metabolism also tends to slow down, making it easier to gain weight and harder to lose it. To overcome this challenge, it is important to focus on maintaining a healthy and balanced diet, as well as incorporating regular cardiovascular exercises into your routine. This can help to boost your metabolism and increase calorie burn, making it easier to achieve and maintain a healthy weight.

By addressing these age-related challenges head-on and incorporating targeted strategies into your fitness routine, you can unleash your potential and continue to live a healthy and active life well into your middle-age and beyond. Remember, age is just a number, and with the right mindset and approach, you can overcome any obstacle that comes your way. So, take charge of your health and fitness journey today, and unlock your true potential after 40!

Finding Support and Accountability

In the journey towards fitness and unleashing your potential after 40, one of the most crucial factors that can make or break your success is finding the right support and accountability. As middle-aged men and women, we often face unique challenges and responsibilities that can make it difficult to prioritize our health and well-being. However, with the right support system and accountability mechanisms in place, we can overcome these obstacles and achieve our fitness goals.

Having a support system is essential in maintaining motivation and staying on track with your fitness journey. Surrounding yourself with like-minded individuals who share similar goals can provide the encouragement and inspiration needed to keep going, even on the toughest days. Seek out fitness communities, join local fitness classes, or find online forums where you can connect with others who are also striving for a healthier lifestyle. By sharing experiences, challenges, and triumphs, you can find solace in knowing that you are not alone in your journey.

Accountability is another crucial element in achieving long-term success. As a fitness and exercise wellness coach, you understand the importance of setting goals and tracking progress. However, it can be challenging to hold yourself accountable, especially when life gets busy. This is where finding an external source of accountability can make all the difference. Consider partnering with a fitness buddy, hiring a personal trainer, or enlisting the support of a wellness coach who can provide guidance, track your progress, and hold you accountable for your actions.

Furthermore, technology can be a valuable tool in finding support and accountability. Numerous fitness apps and online platforms offer features such as goal tracking, meal planning, and community support. These resources can help you stay accountable and provide the necessary support, even when you cannot physically be with others.

Remember, finding support and accountability is not a sign of weakness but rather a strength. It takes courage and determination to acknowledge that you cannot do it alone. By embracing a support system, seeking external accountability, and utilizing technology, you can create a solid foundation for success in your fitness journey.

In conclusion, as middle-aged men and women, finding support and accountability is crucial in our quest for fitness and unleashing our potential after 40. Surround yourself with like-minded individuals, seek external accountability sources, and leverage technology to create a strong support system. With the right support and accountability mechanisms in place, you can overcome challenges, stay motivated, and achieve your fitness goals, ultimately unlocking your true potential.

Staying Motivated in the Long Run

One of the biggest challenges many middle-aged men and women face when it comes to maintaining their fitness and exercise routines is staying motivated in the long run. It's not uncommon to start off with a burst of enthusiasm and dedication, only to find that it fizzles out over time. However, with the right mindset and strategies, you can overcome this hurdle and unleash your potential after 40.

First and foremost, it's important to set realistic and achievable goals. Many people make the mistake of setting lofty targets that are difficult to reach, which can lead to frustration and demotivation. Instead, break your goals down into smaller, more manageable milestones. Celebrate each achievement along the way, as this will give you a sense of accomplishment and keep you motivated to continue.

Another effective way to stay motivated is by finding an exercise routine that you genuinely enjoy. If you dread every workout, it's only a matter of time before you start making excuses to skip them. Try different activities until you find something that brings you joy. Whether it's dancing, swimming, hiking, or joining a sports team, finding an exercise you love will make it easier to stay committed in the long run.

Accountability is another key factor in maintaining motivation. Consider partnering with a fitness and exercise wellness coach who can provide guidance, support, and hold you accountable for your goals. Having someone to answer to and share your progress with can greatly increase your commitment and motivation.

In addition to external accountability, it's important to cultivate self-discipline and develop a routine. Consistency is key when it comes to long-term success in fitness and exercise. Create a schedule that works for you and stick to it. Treat your workouts as non-negotiable appointments with yourself and prioritize them just like you would any other important commitment.

Lastly, remember to celebrate your progress and practice self-compassion. Fitness is a journey, and there will be ups and downs along the way. Don't beat yourself up for the occasional setback or missed workout. Instead, acknowledge your efforts and focus on getting back on track. Surround yourself with positive and supportive individuals who will encourage and motivate you.

By setting realistic goals, finding enjoyable activities, seeking accountability, maintaining discipline, and practicing self-compassion, you can stay motivated in the long run and unleash your potential after 40. Remember, you have the power to achieve your fitness and exercise goals and lead a healthy, fulfilling life at any age.

Chapter 6: Preventing Injuries and Enhancing Recovery

Understanding Common Injuries in Midlife

As we embark on our fitness journey in midlife, it is essential to be aware of the common injuries that can occur during this phase. Our bodies change as we age, and while exercise is crucial for maintaining overall health and well-being, it is important to exercise with caution. By understanding and recognizing these common injuries, we can take necessary precautions and make informed decisions to prevent them.

One of the most prevalent injuries in midlife is joint pain, particularly in the knees and hips. This is often caused by wear and tear on the joints over time, as well as the loss of muscle mass and flexibility. Engaging in weight-bearing exercises and high-impact activities without proper warm-up and stretching can exacerbate these conditions. It is crucial to listen to our bodies and modify exercises to reduce the impact on these vulnerable areas.

Muscle strains and sprains are also common in midlife, especially when we push ourselves too hard or engage in unfamiliar activities. Overexertion or sudden movements can lead to muscle tears or ligament sprains. It is essential to gradually increase the intensity and duration of our workouts, allowing our muscles and connective tissues to adapt and strengthen over time. Proper warm-up and cool-down exercises, as well as incorporating stretching and flexibility routines, can significantly reduce the risk of these injuries.

Back pain is another frequent complaint among middle-aged individuals. Poor posture, weak core muscles, and spinal degeneration are some of the contributing factors. Engaging in exercises that strengthen the core, such as Pilates or yoga, can help alleviate back pain and improve posture. It is important to learn proper lifting techniques and avoid activities that put excessive strain on the back.

Additionally, stress fractures can occur due to repetitive stress on the bones, most commonly in the feet and shins. These injuries can result from activities like running or jumping. Varying our exercise routines and incorporating low-impact activities like swimming or cycling can help reduce the risk of stress fractures.

Understanding these common injuries in midlife is the first step in preventing them. As fitness and exercise wellness coaches, it is crucial to educate middle-aged men and women on these potential risks. By promoting a balanced and tailored approach to exercise, we can help our clients unleash their potential after 40 while minimizing the chance of injury. Remember, fitness is a lifelong journey, and taking care of our bodies is paramount in attaining and maintaining optimal health and well-being.

Injury Prevention Strategies

As we age, the importance of injury prevention becomes even more vital. Our bodies may not be as resilient as they once were, and recovering from an injury can take longer than expected. In this subchapter, we will discuss various strategies that can help middle-aged men and women stay fit and active without putting themselves at risk of injury.

1. Warm-up and cool-down routines: Before starting any exercise, it is crucial to warm up your muscles and joints. This can be done through gentle stretching, light cardiovascular exercises, or even a short walk. Similarly, cooling down after a workout helps your body gradually return to its resting state, reducing the risk of muscle soreness and injury.

2. Proper technique and form: Whether you are lifting weights, performing yoga poses, or participating in a high-intensity workout, using proper technique and form is essential. This ensures that you are engaging the correct muscles, reducing strain on joints, and minimizing the risk of injury. Consider working with a fitness and exercise wellness coach who can guide you in mastering the correct form for each exercise.

3. Gradual progression: It can be tempting to push yourself to the limit when starting a fitness program, but this can lead to overexertion and injury. Instead, focus on gradual progression by gradually increasing the intensity, duration, or frequency of your workouts. This allows your body to adapt and build strength over time, reducing the risk of overuse injuries.

4. Cross-training: Engaging in a variety of exercises and activities is not only beneficial for overall fitness but also helps prevent overuse injuries. Cross-training involves incorporating different types of exercises into your routine, such as cardio, strength training, flexibility exercises, and balance training. This helps to strengthen different muscle groups and reduces the risk of overloading specific areas.

5. Listen to your body: Paying attention to how your body feels during and after exercise is crucial. If you experience pain, discomfort, or notice any unusual sensations, it is important to stop and assess the situation. Pushing through pain can lead to serious injury, so it is better to take a break, modify the exercise, or seek professional advice.

By incorporating these injury prevention strategies into your fitness routine, you can continue to unleash your potential after 40 while minimizing the risk of setbacks. Remember, fitness is a lifelong journey, and taking care of your body is the key to long-term success and overall well-being.

Proper Warm-Up and Cool-Down Techniques

As we age, it becomes increasingly important to take care of our bodies and prioritize our overall health and well-being. Regular exercise and physical activity are essential components of a healthy lifestyle, particularly for middle-aged individuals. To optimize your fitness journey and minimize the risk of injury, it is crucial to incorporate proper warm-up and cool-down techniques into your exercise routine.

The warm-up phase is a vital preparatory step before engaging in any physical activity. It involves gradually increasing your heart rate, blood flow, and body temperature, priming your muscles, joints, and cardiovascular system for exercise. A proper warm-up allows your body to adjust to the increased demands it will face during the workout, reducing the risk of strains, sprains, and other injuries.

Start your warm-up with five to ten minutes of light cardiovascular exercises such as brisk walking, jogging, or cycling. This will gradually elevate your heart rate and increase blood flow to your muscles. Follow this with dynamic stretches that target the major muscle groups you will be using during your workout. Dynamic stretches involve controlled movements that take your joints and muscles through a full range of motion, improving flexibility and enhancing performance.

After completing your workout, it is equally important to cool down properly. The cool-down phase allows your body to gradually return to its resting state, preventing dizziness, muscle soreness, and potential injuries. It also aids in waste removal from your muscles, reducing the likelihood of post-exercise muscle stiffness and cramping.

To cool down effectively, perform five to ten minutes of low-intensity cardiovascular exercise, similar to your warm-up routine. This gentle activity will gradually lower your heart rate and help remove metabolic waste products from your muscles. Follow this with static stretching exercises, holding each stretch for 15-30 seconds, targeting all the major muscle groups you worked during your workout. Static stretching promotes muscle relaxation, flexibility, and reduces muscle tension.

Remember, warm-up and cool-down techniques are not time-consuming, but they are essential for your overall fitness and injury prevention. By incorporating these into your exercise routine, you can unleash your potential after 40, achieving optimal results while minimizing the risk of setbacks. Always consult with a fitness and exercise wellness coach for personalized warm-up and cool-down techniques tailored to your specific needs and abilities. Stay committed to your fitness journey and enjoy the countless benefits that come with taking care of your body.

Recovery Techniques for Optimal Performance

In the pursuit of a healthy and active lifestyle, recovery is often overlooked by many individuals, especially middle-aged men and women. However, understanding the importance of recovery techniques is crucial for achieving optimal performance and unleashing your potential, even after the age of 40. This subchapter will delve into various recovery techniques that will help you stay on top of your fitness game and prevent injuries.

As a fitness and exercise wellness coach, it is essential to educate your clients about the significance of recovery in their fitness journey. Encourage them to prioritize rest and recovery just as much as they prioritize their workouts. By doing so, they will not only enhance their overall performance but also improve their mental focus and reduce the risk of burnout.

One of the most effective recovery techniques is adequate sleep. Middle-aged individuals often struggle with sleep disturbances, which can negatively impact their fitness goals. Encourage your clients to establish a consistent sleep schedule and create a relaxing bedtime routine. Quality sleep is essential for muscle repair, hormone regulation, and mental rejuvenation.

Another crucial aspect of recovery is nutrition. Middle-aged men and women should focus on consuming a well-balanced diet rich in lean proteins, whole grains, fruits, and vegetables. Encourage them to prioritize hydration and avoid excessive consumption of alcohol and processed foods. Adequate nutrition will provide the necessary nutrients for muscle recovery and help maintain a healthy weight.

Additionally, incorporating active recovery days into their exercise routine is crucial. Encourage your clients to engage in low-impact activities such as yoga, swimming, or walking on their recovery days. These activities promote blood circulation, improve flexibility, and reduce muscle soreness.

Furthermore, emphasize the importance of proper stretching and foam rolling to release tension and improve flexibility. Middle-aged individuals may experience tight muscles due to age-related changes or previous injuries. Regular stretching and foam rolling will help alleviate muscle tightness and improve mobility, preventing injuries during workouts.

Lastly, stress management techniques play a pivotal role in recovery. Encourage your clients to practice relaxation techniques such as deep breathing exercises, meditation, or engaging in hobbies they enjoy. Chronic stress can hinder recovery and negatively impact overall health, so it is crucial to address stress management as part of their fitness journey.

By incorporating these recovery techniques into their routine, middle-aged men and women can optimize their performance, prevent injuries, and unleash their potential after 40. As a fitness and exercise wellness coach, it is your role to guide and support them in their journey towards a healthier and more fulfilling life.

Listening to Your Body and Avoiding Overtraining

As we age, it becomes even more crucial to pay attention to our bodies and listen to the signals it sends us during exercise. Overtraining, also known as excessive exercise, can have detrimental effects on our physical and mental well-being. In this subchapter, we will explore the importance of listening to your body and provide strategies to avoid overtraining.

Middle-aged men and women are often caught up in the fast-paced, high-pressure world, where pushing oneself to the limit is seen as a badge of honor. However, it is essential to understand that our bodies have limitations, and ignoring them can lead to injuries, burnout, and a decline in overall fitness.

One of the first steps to avoiding overtraining is to recognize the signs and symptoms. Fatigue, persistent muscle soreness, decreased performance, irritability, and disturbed sleep are all red flags that your body may be on the brink of overtraining. When you notice these signs, it's crucial to take a step back and reassess your exercise routine.

Understanding the concept of periodization is paramount in preventing overtraining. Periodization involves dividing your training into specific phases, with each phase focusing on different goals and intensities. This approach allows for adequate recovery time and prevents overuse injuries. By incorporating periods of lighter training or complete rest, you give your body a chance to recover and adapt, leading to better overall results.

Another key aspect is to prioritize recovery and self-care. Middle-aged individuals often have additional responsibilities and stressors outside of their exercise routine. Taking time to rest, relax, and engage in activities that promote recovery, such as stretching, foam rolling, and massage, can go a long way in preventing overtraining. Adequate sleep and proper nutrition are also critical in supporting your body's recovery process.

Listening to your body also means being mindful of any pain or discomfort during exercise. While it is normal to experience some muscle soreness after a challenging workout, sharp or persistent pain could indicate an injury. Ignoring these warning signs and pushing through the pain can lead to long-term damage. If you experience pain, it is essential to seek professional advice and modify your exercise routine accordingly.

In conclusion, as a fitness and exercise wellness coach, it is crucial to educate middle-aged men and women about the importance of listening to their bodies and avoiding overtraining. By recognizing the signs and symptoms, understanding periodization, prioritizing recovery, and being mindful of pain, individuals can maintain a healthy and sustainable exercise routine. Remember, our bodies are unique, and what works for one person may not work for another. By finding the right balance and listening to our bodies, we can unleash our full potential after 40 and enjoy a lifetime of fitness and well-being.

Chapter 7: Fitness for Life: Aging Gracefully

Embracing the Aging Process

As we journey through life, one thing is certain: we all age. However, instead of fearing the inevitable, it's time to embrace the aging process and unlock our full potential. In this subchapter, we will explore how middle-aged men and women can navigate the challenges and opportunities that come with aging.

Fitness and exercise wellness coach, you hold the key to guiding individuals towards a fulfilling and healthy lifestyle, even in their middle-age years. It's essential to help your clients understand that age is just a number, and with the right mindset and approach, they can continue to thrive physically, mentally, and emotionally.

Physical fitness becomes even more crucial as we age. Encourage your clients to engage in regular exercise, focusing on activities that enhance strength, flexibility, and cardiovascular health. By incorporating a well-rounded fitness routine, individuals can improve their overall well-being, reduce the risk of chronic diseases, and maintain a healthy weight.

It's important to emphasize the significance of adapting exercise routines to accommodate any physical limitations or health conditions that may arise with age. Encourage your clients to listen to their bodies and consult with healthcare professionals to create personalized exercise plans. By doing so, they can prevent injuries and make necessary modifications while still reaping the benefits of physical activity.

Apart from physical fitness, middle-aged men and women must also prioritize their mental and emotional well-being. The aging process may bring about various life changes, such as children leaving the nest, career transitions, or even the loss of loved ones. As a wellness coach, encourage your clients to embrace these changes as opportunities for personal growth and self-discovery.

Support your clients in adopting mindfulness practices such as meditation and stress-reducing techniques. These tools can help individuals manage the complexities of life, reduce anxiety, and promote a positive outlook. Additionally, encourage them to prioritize self-care activities that bring them joy and relaxation, such as hobbies, vacations, or quality time spent with loved ones.

In conclusion, embracing the aging process is about recognizing the limitless potential that lies within each individual, regardless of their age. As a fitness and exercise wellness coach, it is your role to guide middle-aged men and women towards a fulfilling life by encouraging physical fitness, mental well-being, and self-care. By embracing the aging process, your clients can unleash their true potential and live life to the fullest, embracing every stage with grace and vitality.

Adjusting Exercise Routines as You Age

As we age, our bodies undergo various physiological changes that can affect our ability to maintain the same exercise routines we followed in our younger years. However, this doesn't mean we should give up on fitness altogether. In fact, it is crucial to adjust our exercise routines to suit our changing bodies and ensure we continue to lead a healthy and active lifestyle. In this subchapter, we will explore the importance of adjusting exercise routines as we age and provide practical tips for middle-aged men and women to stay fit and strong.

Understanding the Changes

Before diving into specific adjustments, it is essential to understand the changes that occur in our bodies as we age. Our metabolism slows down, muscle mass decreases, bone density declines, and joints become less flexible. These changes can lead to increased risk of injury, decreased endurance, and reduced overall fitness.

Tailoring Your Exercise Routine

When adjusting your exercise routine, it's crucial to focus on three key areas: strength training, cardiovascular exercise, and flexibility training.

Strength Training: As muscle mass naturally declines with age, incorporating strength training exercises is vital to maintaining muscle tone and strength. Opt for weightlifting, resistance bands, or bodyweight exercises to improve muscle strength and prevent muscle loss.

Cardiovascular Exercise: Engaging in aerobic activities like brisk walking, swimming, or cycling can help improve cardiovascular health, maintain a healthy weight, and boost overall fitness levels. However, it's important to listen to your body and choose low-impact exercises to reduce joint stress.

Flexibility Training: Stretching exercises and yoga can help maintain flexibility and prevent stiffness in joints. Regular stretching routines can also aid in reducing the risk of injuries and improving balance.

Additional Considerations

As a middle-aged individual, it is crucial to listen to your body and make adjustments accordingly. Always warm up before exercising, and pay attention to any discomfort or pain during and after the workout. If necessary, consult with a fitness and exercise wellness coach who can provide personalized guidance and tailor an exercise routine to your specific needs.

Remember, it's never too late to start or adjust your exercise routine. Regular physical activity will not only help you maintain a healthy weight, increase energy levels, and improve mood but also reduce the risk of chronic diseases such as heart disease and diabetes.

In conclusion, adjusting exercise routines as we age is essential for maintaining our health and well-being. By understanding the changes that occur in our bodies and making appropriate modifications to our exercise routines, we can continue to unleash our potential and live our best lives well into our middle-aged years and beyond.

Maintaining Cognitive Health Through Fitness

As we age, it's not just our physical health that needs attention, but also our cognitive health. The good news is that staying fit and active can have a profound impact on maintaining cognitive function as we grow older. In this subchapter, we will explore how fitness can benefit your brain and provide practical tips for incorporating exercise into your daily routine.

Exercise has been shown to enhance cognitive function and improve memory and attention span. Regular physical activity increases blood flow to the brain, which promotes the growth of new neurons and strengthens the connections between existing ones. This can result in improved cognitive abilities, such as enhanced problem-solving skills and better decision-making.

Additionally, exercise stimulates the release of chemicals in the brain, such as endorphins and dopamine, which are known to improve mood and reduce stress and anxiety. By reducing these negative factors, fitness plays a vital role in preventing cognitive decline and age-related neurodegenerative diseases, such as Alzheimer's and dementia.

So how can you incorporate fitness into your daily routine to maintain cognitive health? Here are a few practical tips:

1. Engage in aerobic exercise: Activities like brisk walking, jogging, swimming, or cycling increase your heart rate and oxygen flow to the brain, promoting cognitive health.

2. Include strength training: Resistance exercises, such as weightlifting or using resistance bands, not only build muscle but also stimulate brain health by triggering the release of growth factors.

3. Try mind-body exercises: Practices like yoga, tai chi, or Pilates combine physical movement with mental focus, improving cognitive function and reducing stress.

4. Break up sedentary time: If you have a desk job, make a conscious effort to stand up and move around every hour. Even short bursts of physical activity can have a positive impact on your brain health.

5. Challenge your brain: Engage in activities that stimulate your mind, such as puzzles, crosswords, or learning a new language. These mental exercises, combined with physical fitness, can have a synergistic effect on cognitive health.

By prioritizing fitness and exercise, you can unleash your potential and maintain cognitive health well into your middle age and beyond. Remember, it's never too late to start taking care of your brain, and the benefits of a fit and active lifestyle go far beyond physical appearance. So, lace up those sneakers, embrace the power of fitness, and unlock the true potential of your mind.

Promoting Emotional Well-being Through Exercise

In today's fast-paced and stressful world, it is more important than ever to prioritize our emotional well-being. As middle-aged men and women, the demands of work, family, and personal responsibilities can take a toll on our mental health. However, there is a powerful tool that can help us combat stress, anxiety, and depression while improving our overall well-being - exercise.

Exercise has long been recognized for its physical benefits, but its positive impact on our mental health is equally remarkable. Engaging in regular physical activity releases endorphins, the feel-good hormones that boost our mood and reduce stress. Whether it's a brisk walk in the park, a yoga class, or strength training at the gym, any form of exercise can help alleviate symptoms of anxiety and depression.

Additionally, exercise provides an opportunity for self-care and self-reflection. As a fitness and exercise wellness coach, I encourage you to view exercise as a time to connect with yourself and prioritize your needs. This could mean setting aside a designated time each day for exercise, creating a workout routine that suits your preferences and goals, or exploring different types of physical activities that bring you joy.

Furthermore, exercise can be a social outlet, fostering connections and support networks. Joining a group fitness class, participating in team sports, or finding a workout buddy can not only make exercise more enjoyable but also provide a sense of community and belonging. Surrounding yourself with like-minded individuals who share your fitness goals can be incredibly motivating and uplifting.

It is essential to remember that exercise should be approached with a balanced mindset. Rather than focusing solely on the physical outcomes, such as weight loss or muscle gain, prioritize the emotional benefits that exercise brings. Celebrate the small victories, such as feeling energized after a workout or noticing an improvement in your mood. Embrace the journey and focus on progress, not perfection.

In conclusion, promoting emotional well-being through exercise is a powerful tool for middle-aged men and women seeking to enhance their overall quality of life. As a fitness and exercise wellness coach, I encourage you to make exercise a priority in your daily routine, not only for its physical benefits but also for the positive impact it can have on your mental health. Embrace the opportunity for self-care, use exercise as a social outlet, and celebrate the emotional victories along the way. By unleashing your potential through exercise, you can achieve a healthier and happier life after 40.

Integrating Fitness into Everyday Life

In today's fast-paced world, where work and family commitments often take precedence, finding time for fitness can be a challenge. However, incorporating exercise into your daily routine is essential, especially as we age. This subchapter aims to provide middle-aged men and women with practical strategies for integrating fitness into their everyday lives, empowering them to unleash their potential and prioritize their health and well-being.

One of the most effective ways to integrate fitness into your daily routine is by making small, incremental changes. Start by incorporating physical activity into activities you already enjoy. For example, instead of meeting friends for coffee, suggest going for a walk together. By combining socializing with exercise, you can make fitness a more enjoyable and sustainable part of your life.

Another key strategy is to find pockets of time throughout your day where you can sneak in some physical activity. This could be as simple as taking the stairs instead of the elevator, parking your car farther away from your destination, or doing a quick workout during your lunch break. By seizing these opportunities, you can accumulate exercise minutes without disrupting your busy schedule.

Furthermore, setting tangible goals can provide the motivation and structure necessary to stay on track. Whether it's signing up for a local 5K race, aiming to do a certain number of push-ups, or striving to walk a certain distance each day, having a clear target can help you stay focused and committed to your fitness journey.

Additionally, seeking the guidance of a fitness and exercise wellness coach can be invaluable. These professionals are trained to create personalized fitness programs that cater to your specific needs and goals. They can also provide valuable accountability and support, ensuring that you stay motivated and on track.

Remember, integrating fitness into your everyday life is not about perfection. It's about finding realistic and sustainable ways to prioritize your health. By making small changes, seizing opportunities for physical activity, setting goals, and seeking professional guidance, you can unleash your potential and enjoy a healthier and more fulfilling life after 40.

So, let's take the first step towards integrating fitness into our everyday lives and embark on this transformative journey together. Your body and mind will thank you for it!

Chapter 8: Taking Your Fitness to the Next Level

Exploring Advanced Training Techniques

In the pursuit of optimal fitness and wellness, it is crucial to continually challenge and push ourselves beyond our comfort zones. This is especially true for middle-aged men and women who are looking to unleash their potential and achieve their fitness goals. In this subchapter, we will delve into the world of advanced training techniques that can take your fitness journey to the next level.

1. High-Intensity Interval Training (HIIT):
HIIT workouts involve alternating between short bursts of intense exercise and brief recovery periods. This technique not only boosts cardiovascular endurance but also enhances fat burning and improves overall fitness levels. With HIIT, you can maximize your workout in less time, making it ideal for busy individuals.

2. Strength Training:
Strength training is a key component of any fitness routine, particularly for middle-aged individuals seeking to preserve muscle mass and bone density. Advanced techniques such as supersets, drop sets, and pyramid training can help to challenge your muscles and stimulate growth, leading to improved strength and a toned physique.

3. Plyometrics:
Plyometric exercises involve explosive movements that rapidly stretch and contract muscles, improving power and agility. Incorporating exercises like box jumps, medicine ball throws, and jump squats can enhance athletic performance and overall functional fitness.

4. Suspension Training:

Suspension training utilizes straps and bodyweight exercises to build strength, stability, and flexibility. This technique engages multiple muscle groups simultaneously and can be easily adapted to all fitness levels. By incorporating suspension training into your routine, you can improve core strength, balance, and overall muscular endurance.

5. Yoga and Pilates Fusion:

Combining the principles of yoga and Pilates can provide a well-rounded approach to fitness and wellness. This fusion technique emphasizes flexibility, core strength, and mindfulness, offering numerous benefits such as improved posture, reduced stress, and enhanced mind-body connection.

It is important to note that before incorporating these advanced training techniques into your fitness routine, it is advisable to consult a fitness and exercise wellness coach. They can provide personalized guidance, help you set realistic goals, and ensure you are performing exercises correctly to prevent injuries.

Remember, as middle-aged individuals, our bodies may require more recovery time between workouts. Listen to your body, stay consistent, and gradually increase the intensity of your workouts to avoid burnout and achieve long-term success.

By embracing advanced training techniques, you can unleash your potential and embark on a transformative fitness journey that will not only improve your physical well-being but also enhance your overall quality of life.

Participating in Competitive Events

For middle-aged men and women who are seeking to enhance their fitness journey, participating in competitive events can be an exhilarating and rewarding experience. Whether you are an avid fitness enthusiast or someone who is just starting out on their wellness journey, competitive events provide an excellent opportunity to challenge yourself, set new goals, and unleash your potential after 40.

Competitive events come in various forms, ranging from local 5K races to triathlons, obstacle course races, and even bodybuilding competitions. Engaging in these events not only helps you stay motivated and committed to your fitness routine but also allows you to connect with like-minded individuals and build a sense of camaraderie within the fitness community.

One of the key benefits of participating in competitive events is the opportunity to set new goals and push your limits. These events provide a tangible target to work towards, giving you a sense of purpose and direction in your fitness journey. Whether your goal is to finish a race, improve your personal best, or simply enjoy the experience, competitive events provide a structured platform to strive for continuous improvement.

Moreover, competitive events promote a healthy competitive spirit that can fuel your motivation and drive. They encourage you to step out of your comfort zone, challenge yourself physically and mentally, and overcome obstacles along the way. By embracing these events, you can cultivate resilience, discipline, and determination – qualities that are not only beneficial in the fitness realm but also in various aspects of your life.

As a fitness and exercise wellness coach, I strongly recommend participating in competitive events to my clients. These events provide an opportunity to showcase the progress you have made and celebrate your achievements. It is important to remember that competitive events are not solely about winning; they are about personal growth, self-improvement, and having fun along the way.

Before participating in any competitive event, it is essential to prepare adequately. Engage in a well-rounded training program that includes cardiovascular exercises, strength training, and flexibility work to ensure you are adequately conditioned. Additionally, consult with a qualified fitness professional or coach who can guide you through the process and help you set realistic goals.

In conclusion, participating in competitive events can be an empowering and fulfilling experience for middle-aged men and women on their fitness journey. These events provide an avenue to challenge yourself, set new goals, and unleash your potential. Embrace the opportunity, push your limits, and enjoy the thrill of being part of the competitive fitness community. Remember, the journey is just as important as the destination.

Setting New Challenges and Goals

In the journey of life, it is essential to constantly set new challenges and goals for ourselves. This holds especially true for middle-aged men and women who are seeking to maintain their fitness and unleash their potential after the age of 40. As a fitness and exercise wellness coach, I understand the importance of continuously pushing our limits and striving for new achievements. In this subchapter, we will delve into the significance of setting new challenges and goals and how it can contribute to your overall well-being.

As we age, our bodies go through various changes, both physically and mentally. However, it is crucial not to let these changes hinder our progress towards a healthier and happier lifestyle. By setting new challenges and goals, we can overcome obstacles and break through limitations that may have previously held us back. This process not only helps us improve our physical fitness but also boosts our mental resilience and confidence.

One of the key benefits of setting new challenges and goals is that it keeps us motivated and focused. Whether it is aiming to run a marathon, mastering a new yoga pose, or increasing your strength in the gym, having a specific target in mind gives us something to work towards. This sense of purpose and direction can be immensely empowering and helps us maintain our dedication to our overall fitness and wellness journey.

Additionally, setting new challenges and goals provides us with opportunities for personal growth and self-discovery. It forces us to step out of our comfort zones and explore new territories. By trying new exercises or engaging in different fitness activities, we can discover hidden talents, passions, and interests that we may not have known existed. This process of self-discovery can be incredibly fulfilling and can lead to a more enriched and purposeful life.

However, it is important to approach these challenges and goals with a realistic mindset. It is crucial to set attainable targets and not overwhelm ourselves with unrealistic expectations. By breaking down our goals into smaller, manageable steps, we can ensure steady progress and avoid burnout or disappointment.

In conclusion, setting new challenges and goals is a crucial aspect of unleashing your potential after 40. As a fitness and exercise wellness coach, I encourage all middle-aged men and women to embrace new challenges and set meaningful goals. It is through these endeavors that we can push our limits, discover our true potential, and lead a healthier, happier, and more fulfilling life.

Exploring Different Fitness Modalities

In the quest for a healthy and fulfilling life, it is essential to explore various fitness modalities that can unlock your potential, especially as a middle-aged individual. This subchapter aims to provide valuable insights into different fitness options and their benefits, specifically tailored to the needs of middle-aged men and women. Whether you are a fitness enthusiast, exercise wellness coach, or someone looking to improve their overall well-being, this section will guide you towards finding the most suitable fitness modality for your individual goals.

1. Strength Training: As we age, maintaining muscle mass becomes increasingly important. Strength training not only helps prevent muscle loss but also improves bone density and overall strength. This modality can be customized according to your fitness level, allowing you to gradually increase the intensity and challenge yourself.

2. Cardiovascular Exercise: Engaging in regular cardiovascular exercise is vital for heart health and weight management. From brisk walking and jogging to swimming and cycling, there are numerous options available to get your heart pumping. This section will explore various cardiovascular exercises and provide tips on how to incorporate them into your daily routine.

3. Yoga and Pilates: Middle-aged individuals often experience joint stiffness and reduced flexibility. Yoga and Pilates are excellent modalities to address these concerns. Both practices focus on strengthening the core, improving posture, and increasing flexibility. This subchapter will delve into the benefits of these mind-body exercises, along with tips for beginners.

4. Functional Training: Maintaining functional fitness is crucial as we age. Functional training exercises mimic movements we perform in our daily lives, enhancing our ability to perform everyday tasks with ease. This section will discuss exercises that target balance, coordination, and mobility, ensuring that you stay active and independent as you age.

5. Mindfulness and Meditation: Fitness is not limited to physical activity alone; it also encompasses mental well-being. Mindfulness and meditation practices can help reduce stress, improve focus, and promote overall mental health. This subchapter will explore different techniques to incorporate mindfulness and meditation into your fitness routine.

By exploring these different fitness modalities, you can create a well-rounded exercise regimen that caters to your individual needs as a middle-aged man or woman. Remember, it is essential to consult with a fitness and exercise wellness coach to ensure you are performing exercises correctly and maximizing your potential. So, let's embark on this journey of self-discovery and unleash your true fitness potential after 40!

Inspiring Others and Becoming a Fitness Advocate

As we embark on our journey towards health and wellness, we often find inspiration from those who have overcome obstacles and achieved great success in their fitness endeavors. In this subchapter, we will explore the importance of inspiring others and becoming a fitness advocate, specifically addressing the middle-aged men and women in our audience who are fitness and exercise wellness coaches.

Middle age is a critical time when many individuals may feel discouraged or overwhelmed by the physical changes that come with aging. However, it is also a time when we can make significant positive changes in our lives, both physically and mentally. As fitness advocates, we have the power to motivate and inspire others to embrace a healthier lifestyle and unleash their potential after 40.

One of the most effective ways to inspire others is by leading by example. As fitness and exercise wellness coaches, it is essential to prioritize our own health and well-being. When others see our dedication and commitment to fitness, it becomes easier for them to envision themselves making similar changes. By sharing our own personal journeys, challenges, and triumphs, we can create a sense of relatability and authenticity that resonates with our audience.

Furthermore, as fitness advocates, we have the opportunity to educate and inform through various platforms. Whether it be through social media, blogs, or public speaking engagements, we can provide valuable insights, practical tips, and evidence-based information to help middle-aged men and women navigate their fitness journeys.

Additionally, building a supportive community is crucial to inspiring others. Creating a safe and welcoming space where individuals can share their experiences, ask questions, and receive guidance is essential. By fostering a sense of belonging and camaraderie, we can empower others to take charge of their health and fitness.

Finally, it is important to celebrate the successes of those we inspire. By acknowledging and recognizing their accomplishments, we not only boost their confidence but also encourage others to follow in their footsteps. By highlighting real-life stories of middle-aged men and women who have transformed their lives through fitness, we can inspire others to take action and make positive changes of their own.

In conclusion, as fitness and exercise wellness coaches, we have the power to inspire and motivate middle-aged men and women to embrace a healthier lifestyle. By leading by example, sharing our personal journeys, providing valuable information, fostering a supportive community, and celebrating successes, we can become powerful advocates for fitness and unleash the potential of those around us. Let us come together and inspire others to embark on their own transformative fitness journeys, unlocking a world of possibilities after 40.

Chapter 9: Creating a Sustainable Fitness Lifestyle

Building Long-Term Habits

In order to unleash your potential and achieve optimal fitness and wellness after 40, it is crucial to focus on building long-term habits. Developing consistent routines and healthy lifestyle choices will not only benefit your physical health but also contribute to your overall well-being. This subchapter will guide you through the process of building long-term habits and help you stay committed to your fitness goals.

1. Set Clear Goals: Before embarking on your fitness journey, it is important to establish clear and achievable goals. Whether it is losing weight, improving cardiovascular endurance, or building strength, having a specific target will provide you with motivation and direction.

2. Start Small and Progress Gradually: Rome wasn't built in a day, and neither will your fitness habits. Begin by incorporating small changes into your daily routine. For example, start with a 15-minute walk every morning and gradually increase the duration and intensity as your body adapts. Slow and steady progress is key to avoiding burnout and injuries.

3. Find an Accountability Partner: Having an accountability partner, such as a fitness and exercise wellness coach, can significantly increase your chances of success. They can provide guidance, support, and motivation, ensuring you stay on track and don't give up when faced with challenges.

4. Create a Schedule: Treat your fitness routine like any other important appointment in your calendar. Dedicate specific time slots for exercise and stick to them. By making exercise a non-negotiable part of your daily routine, it becomes easier to build a habit.

5. Make it Enjoyable: Find physical activities that you genuinely enjoy. Whether it's dancing, swimming, hiking, or playing a sport, incorporating activities that bring you joy will make it easier to stay consistent. Experiment with different forms of exercise until you discover what resonates with you the most.

6. Celebrate Milestones: Acknowledge and celebrate your achievements along the way. Each milestone, no matter how small, is a testament to your dedication and hard work. Reward yourself with something meaningful as a way to reinforce the positive habit you've built.

7. Embrace Flexibility: Life is unpredictable, and there will be times when your fitness routine gets disrupted. Embrace flexibility and adaptability. Rather than giving up entirely, find creative ways to stay active during busy periods or when traveling.

Remember, building long-term habits takes time and effort, but the rewards are immeasurable. By implementing these strategies and staying committed to your fitness goals, you can unleash your potential and enjoy a fit and healthy life well beyond your 40s.

Developing a Positive Mindset Towards Fitness

In order to truly unleash your potential and achieve optimal fitness after 40, it is essential to develop a positive mindset towards fitness. Middle-aged men and women often face unique challenges when it comes to maintaining their health and wellness, but with the right mindset, these obstacles can be overcome. This subchapter aims to guide you in cultivating a positive mindset, enabling you to embrace fitness as a lifelong journey.

1. Embrace a Growth Mindset: Recognize that fitness is not a destination but a continuous process. Embrace the belief that you can improve, grow, and overcome any obstacles that come your way. Rather than fixating on past failures or setbacks, focus on the progress you have made and set new goals to keep moving forward.

2. Shift Your Perspective: Instead of viewing exercise as a chore, reframe it as an opportunity for self-care and personal growth. Understand that investing time and effort in your physical well-being will have far-reaching positive effects on your overall quality of life. See exercise as a gift you give yourself, rather than a burden to bear.

3. Celebrate Small Victories: Acknowledge and celebrate every small win along your fitness journey. Whether it's completing an extra rep, running a little longer, or simply showing up consistently, these achievements add up and contribute to your overall progress. By acknowledging and celebrating these victories, you reinforce a positive mindset and build momentum for future successes.

4. Surround Yourself with Positivity: Surround yourself with like-minded individuals who share your commitment to fitness and exercise. Seek out the support of a fitness and exercise wellness coach who can provide guidance, motivation, and accountability. Engaging with a supportive community will help you stay motivated and maintain a positive mindset.

5. Practice Gratitude: Cultivate a sense of gratitude for your body's capabilities and the opportunity to engage in physical activity. Expressing gratitude for the ability to move, breathe, and challenge yourself physically can have a profound impact on your mindset. Gratitude enhances your overall well-being, making fitness an even more rewarding experience.

By developing a positive mindset towards fitness, middle-aged men and women can unlock their full potential and achieve optimal health and wellness. Remember, fitness is not just about physical transformation; it is a journey of self-discovery, personal growth, and empowerment. Embrace the process, celebrate your progress, and let your positive mindset guide you towards a vibrant and fulfilling life.

Finding Joy in Physical Activity

Physical activity is not just about staying fit and maintaining a healthy weight; it is also about finding joy and fulfillment in the process. As we age, it becomes increasingly important to prioritize our physical well-being and engage in activities that bring us happiness. In this subchapter, we will explore how middle-aged men and women can discover and embrace the joy of physical activity.

1. Discovering Your Passion:
Finding joy in physical activity starts with discovering activities that genuinely excite you. It could be anything from dancing, swimming, hiking, or even joining a local sports team. Experiment with different activities until you find something that not only challenges your body but also brings a smile to your face.

2. Setting Realistic Goals:
Setting realistic goals is crucial when it comes to finding joy in physical activity. Instead of focusing solely on weight loss or muscle gain, set goals that are centered around personal growth and achievement. For example, aim to complete a 10K race, master a new yoga pose, or improve your golf swing. These milestones will not only provide a sense of accomplishment but will also make the journey enjoyable.

3. Finding Social Connections:
Physical activity can be even more enjoyable when shared with others. Look for opportunities to engage in group activities or join fitness classes where you can meet like-minded individuals. Having a support system and building social connections can significantly enhance the joy of physical activity.

4. Incorporating Variety:

Monotony can quickly drain the joy out of any physical activity routine. Keep things exciting by incorporating variety into your workouts. Try different exercise modalities, alternate between indoor and outdoor activities, or participate in fitness challenges. By continuously challenging yourself with new experiences, you will stay motivated and find joy in the process.

5. Celebrating Milestones:

Celebrate your achievements along the way to maintain your enthusiasm for physical activity. Whether it's reaching a personal best, overcoming a fitness obstacle, or simply sticking to your exercise routine for a month, take the time to acknowledge and celebrate your accomplishments. Rewarding yourself will reinforce positive behavior and keep the joy alive.

Remember, finding joy in physical activity is a personal journey. Embrace the activities that resonate with you, set realistic goals, find social connections, incorporate variety, and celebrate your achievements. By doing so, you will not only improve your physical health but also unleash your potential for a happier, more fulfilled life after 40.

Incorporating Fitness into Social Interactions

As we navigate through our middle age, it becomes increasingly important to prioritize our health and well-being. Regular exercise and staying active not only contribute to maintaining a healthy weight and physical fitness, but they also have a profound impact on our mental and emotional well-being. In this subchapter, we will explore the significance of incorporating fitness into our social interactions and how it can help us unleash our potential after 40.

For many middle-aged men and women, finding the motivation to exercise can be challenging. However, by incorporating fitness into social interactions, we can transform our exercise routines into enjoyable and engaging activities. Engaging in physical activities with friends, family, or even a fitness and exercise wellness coach can provide the much-needed motivation and accountability to stick to our fitness goals.

One way to incorporate fitness into social interactions is by joining a group exercise class. Whether it's a high-energy Zumba class, a challenging spin class, or a rejuvenating yoga session, group exercise classes offer an opportunity to meet like-minded individuals who share a passion for fitness. Not only will you get your heart pumping and muscles working, but you'll also have the chance to make new friends and build a supportive fitness community.

Another great way to combine fitness with social interactions is by participating in team sports or recreational activities. Joining a local basketball, soccer, or volleyball team not only provides an outlet for physical activity but also fosters teamwork, camaraderie, and healthy competition. You'll not only improve your fitness but also build lasting friendships and create memories that will keep you motivated to stay active.

Additionally, hiring a fitness and exercise wellness coach can be a game-changer for middle-aged men and women. A coach can provide personalized guidance, support, and motivation, ensuring you stay on track with your fitness goals. Moreover, working with a coach can help you build a strong support system and connect with others who are on a similar journey towards better health and well-being.

Incorporating fitness into social interactions is a powerful way to stay motivated, accountable, and inspired on your fitness journey. It not only enhances our physical health but also improves our mental and emotional well-being. By embracing social interactions as a means to incorporate fitness into our lives, we can unleash our potential after 40 and achieve a healthier, happier, and more fulfilling life.

Adapting to Life Changes and Maintaining Consistency

Life is full of changes, and as we age, these changes may become more frequent and sometimes challenging to navigate. For middle-aged men and women, adapting to these changes and maintaining consistency in our fitness and exercise routines becomes crucial for unleashing our potential and leading a fulfilling life. This subchapter explores various strategies and tips to help you adapt to life changes while staying committed to your fitness goals.

One of the key aspects of adapting to life changes is accepting that change is inevitable. Embracing change allows us to move forward and find new opportunities for growth. Whether it's a career change, becoming an empty-nester, or dealing with health issues, understanding that change is a natural part of life will help you maintain a positive mindset and stay motivated.

Consistency is the key to achieving long-term fitness goals. However, life changes can disrupt our routines and make it challenging to stay consistent. In such situations, it's essential to be flexible and adapt your exercise routine to fit your new circumstances. This might mean adjusting your workout schedule, finding alternative exercise options, or seeking the guidance of a fitness and exercise wellness coach.

Maintaining consistency also requires setting realistic goals. As middle-aged individuals, we may have different fitness capabilities and limitations compared to our younger selves. Accepting and embracing these changes will help you set achievable goals that align with your current physical condition. A fitness and exercise wellness coach can play a vital role in helping you set realistic goals and design a workout plan tailored to your specific needs.

Additionally, building a support system is crucial to maintaining consistency and adapting to life changes. Surrounding yourself with like-minded individuals who understand and support your fitness journey can provide motivation, accountability, and a sense of belonging. Joining fitness communities, participating in group workouts, or even seeking the guidance of a fitness and exercise wellness coach can help you build a solid support network.

Lastly, it's important to prioritize self-care and listen to your body. As we age, recovery becomes more critical, and pushing ourselves beyond our limits can lead to injuries or burnout. Incorporating rest days, proper nutrition, and stress management techniques into your routine will ensure that you can adapt to life changes while maintaining consistency and taking care of your overall well-being.

In conclusion, adapting to life changes and maintaining consistency in our fitness and exercise routines is crucial for middle-aged men and women. Embracing change, setting realistic goals, building a support system, and prioritizing self-care are essential strategies to successfully navigate life changes and unleash our potential after 40. With the guidance of a fitness and exercise wellness coach, you can overcome challenges, stay committed to your goals, and lead a healthy and fulfilling life.

Chapter 10: Celebrating Your Fitness Journey

Reflecting on Your Progress and Achievements

In your journey towards fitness and unleashing your potential after 40, it is crucial to take a moment and reflect on your progress and achievements. This subchapter will guide you through the importance of self-reflection and provide you with effective strategies to acknowledge and celebrate your milestones.

Middle-aged men and women, like yourself, often overlook their accomplishments due to the constant focus on future goals. However, taking the time to reflect on how far you have come can be incredibly motivating and inspiring. It allows you to appreciate the hard work and dedication you have put into your fitness journey.

One of the key benefits of reflecting on your progress is gaining a sense of empowerment. Witnessing your achievements firsthand can boost your confidence and self-belief, propelling you forward towards even greater success. By acknowledging the positive changes in your physical abilities, body composition, and overall well-being, you reinforce the notion that you are capable of accomplishing your goals.

To effectively reflect on your progress, start by setting aside dedicated time for self-evaluation. Find a quiet and comfortable space where you can focus without distractions. Begin by reviewing your initial goals and objectives. Have you made progress towards them? What actions have you taken to get where you are today? Take note of any obstacles you overcame along the way and how you managed to overcome them.

Next, consider the physical changes you have noticed in your body. Maybe you have lost weight, gained muscle mass, improved your cardiovascular endurance, or increased your flexibility. Celebrate these achievements and take pride in the hard work you have invested in your fitness and exercise routine.

Another valuable aspect of reflecting on your progress is recognizing the mental and emotional growth you have experienced. Have you developed a more positive mindset? Do you feel more energized, focused, and motivated in your daily life? These non-physical changes are just as important as the physical ones and should be acknowledged and celebrated.

Lastly, don't forget to reward yourself for your achievements. Treat yourself to something special, whether it's a relaxing massage, a new workout outfit, or a weekend getaway. By celebrating your milestones, you reinforce the positive behaviors and habits that have gotten you this far and encourage yourself to keep pushing forward.

In conclusion, reflecting on your progress and achievements is a vital part of your fitness journey after 40. It allows you to appreciate how far you have come, boosts your confidence, and reinforces your belief in your own potential. Take the time to evaluate your goals, acknowledge your physical and mental progress, and reward yourself for your achievements. By doing so, you will continue to unleash your potential and lead a fit and fulfilling life.

Recognizing the Positive Impact of Fitness

In our fast-paced and demanding world, it can be easy to overlook the importance of fitness and its positive impact on our lives. As middle-aged men and women, we often find ourselves juggling multiple responsibilities, leaving little time for self-care. However, understanding and recognizing the profound benefits that fitness can bring to our lives is essential for unleashing our true potential.

Physical fitness not only helps us maintain a healthy weight and prevent chronic diseases, but it also plays a vital role in our mental and emotional well-being. Regular exercise releases endorphins, also known as the "feel-good" hormones, which can boost our mood, reduce stress, and improve our overall mental health. As fitness and exercise wellness coaches, we understand the importance of these factors in maintaining a balanced and fulfilling lifestyle.

Moreover, engaging in regular physical activity can significantly enhance our cognitive abilities. Research has shown that exercise improves memory, focus, and creativity, making it an invaluable tool for middle-aged individuals who are often faced with the challenges of career advancement and personal growth. By recognizing the positive impact of fitness, we can harness its potential to help us excel in all areas of our lives.

Additionally, fitness can greatly improve our energy levels and overall vitality. As we age, we may find ourselves becoming more fatigued and lacking the stamina we once had. However, incorporating regular exercise into our routines can reverse this trend, helping us regain our youthful vigor. By maintaining a consistent fitness regimen, we can experience increased energy, improved sleep quality, and a higher level of overall vitality.

Finally, fitness provides an opportunity for personal growth and self-discovery. Engaging in physical activities challenges us to push beyond our comfort zones, helping us build resilience, determination, and confidence. As fitness and exercise wellness coaches, we are passionate about guiding middle-aged men and women on this transformative journey of self-improvement.

In conclusion, recognizing the positive impact of fitness is crucial for middle-aged individuals seeking to unleash their potential. By incorporating regular physical activity into our lives, we can experience improved mental and emotional well-being, enhanced cognitive abilities, increased energy levels, and personal growth. As fitness and exercise wellness coaches, we are here to support and guide you on this empowering path towards a healthier and more fulfilling life.

Setting New Goals for Continued Growth

As we embark on the journey of life after 40, it is essential for both middle-aged men and women to set new goals for continued growth in their fitness and overall wellness. This subchapter aims to guide and inspire individuals in the niches of fitness and exercise wellness coaching to unleash their potential and embrace a healthy lifestyle.

Reaching the age of 40 is a significant milestone, and it is crucial to acknowledge that our bodies go through natural changes. However, this is not a reason to give up on our fitness goals. Instead, it is an opportunity to set new goals that align with our current stage of life and physical abilities.

First and foremost, it is essential to assess our current fitness levels and identify areas of improvement. This could involve consulting with a fitness and exercise wellness coach who can provide expert guidance tailored to our individual needs. By understanding our strengths and weaknesses, we can set realistic and achievable goals that will contribute to our overall growth.

One crucial aspect of setting new goals is to ensure they are specific, measurable, attainable, relevant, and time-bound (SMART). For example, rather than aiming to "get fit," a specific goal could be to participate in a 5K run within the next six months. This provides a clear target to work towards and helps track progress along the way.

Furthermore, it is important to diversify our fitness routine and incorporate various forms of exercise. This not only prevents monotony but also allows us to target different muscle groups and improve overall strength and flexibility. A fitness and exercise wellness coach can help us explore different activities, such as yoga, swimming, weightlifting, or even martial arts, based on our interests and abilities.

In addition to physical goals, it is equally important to set goals related to nutrition and mental well-being. Middle-aged men and women can benefit from adopting a balanced diet that provides the necessary nutrients while promoting overall health. Moreover, practicing mindfulness techniques, such as meditation or journaling, can enhance mental clarity and reduce stress.

By setting new goals for continued growth, middle-aged men and women can embark on a fulfilling journey towards a healthier and more vibrant life. Remember, it is never too late to unleash your potential and achieve the fitness and wellness you desire. So, let's take the first step towards a better future and embrace the opportunities that lie ahead.

Inspiring Others Through Your Transformation

Subchapter: Inspiring Others Through Your Transformation

In our journey towards a healthier and fitter life, we often forget the immense impact our personal transformation can have on those around us. As middle-aged men and women, we possess the power to inspire and motivate others with our own fitness success stories. This subchapter delves into the significance of sharing our transformational journeys and how we can become beacons of inspiration for others.

1. The Ripple Effect of Transformation:
When we take charge of our physical and mental well-being, we create a ripple effect that extends far beyond ourselves. As fitness and exercise wellness coaches, we can inspire others to embrace a healthier lifestyle, showing them that it's never too late to make positive changes. By sharing our own transformational stories, we empower others to believe in their own potential..

2. Authenticity and Vulnerability:
To truly inspire others, we must be authentic and vulnerable in sharing our journey. Middle age often brings with it unique challenges, such as hormonal changes, increased responsibilities, and a hectic lifestyle. By openly discussing these obstacles and how we overcame them, we show others that they are not alone in their struggles. Our vulnerability allows them to relate and find the strength to start their own transformative journey.

3. Leading by Example:

As fitness and exercise wellness coaches, we have the opportunity to lead by example. By maintaining our own fitness routine and prioritizing our well-being, we demonstrate the importance of self-care. We become living proof that age is just a number and that it's never too late to achieve our goals. Middle-aged men and women who witness our commitment and dedication will be inspired to take action themselves.

4. Building a Supportive Community:

Our transformation can also serve as a catalyst for building a supportive community of like-minded individuals. By sharing our experiences, we can connect with others who are also on a journey towards improved fitness and well-being. Together, we can uplift and motivate each other, creating a network of support that fosters growth and transformation for everyone involved.

5. Inspiring the Next Generation:

By embracing fitness and unleashing our potential after 40, we become role models for future generations. Our children, grandchildren, and even friends' children observe our dedication and perseverance. We show them that aging doesn't mean giving up on our dreams or settling for mediocrity. We inspire them to live a life of vitality and health, setting the stage for a brighter and more active future.

In conclusion, our personal fitness transformation holds the power to inspire others in ways we may never fully comprehend. By sharing our journey with authenticity, leading by example, and building a supportive community, we ignite a spark of motivation in middle-aged men and women who may have once believed that change was impossible. Our transformative stories have the potential to create a ripple effect that extends far beyond ourselves, inspiring others to take control of their own well-being and unleash their untapped potential.

Embracing Fitness as a Lifelong Journey

In our fast-paced and demanding world, it is crucial for middle-aged men and women to prioritize their health and well-being. As we age, our bodies undergo numerous changes, making it even more important to embrace fitness as a lifelong journey. In this subchapter, we will explore the benefits and strategies for staying fit and healthy as we age.

Fitness is not a destination; it is a continuous journey that requires commitment and dedication. As a fitness and exercise wellness coach, I have witnessed countless individuals transform their lives by adopting a proactive approach to their health. This subchapter aims to inspire and guide you to unleash your potential after 40.

One of the key benefits of embracing fitness as a lifelong journey is the preservation of physical and mental health. Regular exercise has been proven to reduce the risk of chronic diseases such as heart disease, diabetes, and certain types of cancer. Additionally, it helps maintain a healthy weight, improves mood, and enhances cognitive function.

To embark on this lifelong journey, it is important to set realistic and achievable goals. Start by assessing your current fitness level and consult with a professional if needed. Consider incorporating a variety of exercises that focus on strength, cardiovascular health, flexibility, and balance. This well-rounded approach will ensure that you address all aspects of your fitness and reduce the risk of injury.

Another vital aspect of this journey is nutrition. As we age, our bodies require different nutrients to support optimal health. It is essential to fuel your body with a balanced diet that includes lean proteins, whole grains, fruits, and vegetables. Stay hydrated and limit processed foods, excess sugar, and unhealthy fats.

Moreover, it is important to remember that fitness is not just about physical exercise; it encompasses mental and emotional well-being as well. Incorporate stress management techniques such as meditation, yoga, or deep breathing exercises into your routine. Take time to relax and prioritize self-care activities that promote mental clarity and emotional stability.

Lastly, remember that fitness is a journey, and setbacks may occur. Do not get discouraged by obstacles along the way. Instead, view them as opportunities for growth and learning. Surround yourself with a supportive community, whether it be friends, family, or a fitness group, to stay motivated and accountable.

In conclusion, embracing fitness as a lifelong journey is essential for middle-aged men and women. By prioritizing our health and adopting a proactive approach, we can unlock our true potential after 40. Remember to set realistic goals, nourish your body with a balanced diet, and prioritize mental and emotional well-being. With dedication and perseverance, this journey will lead to a healthier and more fulfilling life.

www.ingramcontent.com/pod-product-compliance
Lightning Source LLC
Chambersburg PA
CBHW080939260726
48661CB00010B/3997